Personal Medical Services Pilots

Modernising primary care?

Personal Medical Services Pilots

Modernising primary care?

Edited by Richard Lewis, Stephen Gillam
and Clare Jenkins

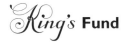

Published by
King's Fund Publishing
11–13 Cavendish Square
London W1G 0AN

© King's Fund 2001

First published 2001

ISBN 1 85717 452 6

A CIP catalogue record for this book is available from the British Library

Available from:
King's Fund Bookshop
11–13 Cavendish Square
London
W1G 0AN

Tel: 020 7307 2591
Fax: 020 7307 2801

Printed and bound in Great Britain

Cover design: Vertigo Design Consultants

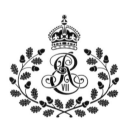

Contents

Contributors

Catherine Baraniak is an independent nurse contractor currently consolidating the nurse-led Meadowfields Practice in Chellaston, Derby.

Tim Crossley is a GP in Wolverhampton and is clinical director of the network of ten salaried GPs employed by the local community trust.

Lance Gardner is an independent nurse clinician leading the Daruzzaman Care Centre in Salford.

Stephen Gillam is Programme Director for Primary Care at the King's Fund.

Clare Jenkins is Project Officer for Personal Medical Services Pilots at the King's Fund.

James Kingsland is senior partner in a first wave PMS pilot in Wallasey and a medical advisor to the Department of Health.

Richard Lewis is a Visiting Fellow in Primary Care at the King's Fund.

Rigo Pizarro-Duhart is Head of Primary Care Contracts at East London and The City Health Authority. For ten years he worked for Lambeth, Southwark and Lewisham Health Authority in the area of primary care contracting and development.

Tim Richardson is a partner in a large dual site practice in Epsom, Surrey, with a keen interest in the development of health care.

Andrew Roscoe is general manager of a large practice, with many years' experience in primary care and the commissioning of hospital services.

Foreword

David Colin-Thomé

The King's Fund is one of the UK's leading authorities on primary care, and has been at the forefront in charting the progress of personal medical services (PMS) pilots.

This evaluation demonstrates the gains and some of the problems inherent in any new initiative. PMS pilots are one of a range of options for primary care, such as local development schemes (LDS) and traditional general medical services (GMS), which offer new ways of benefiting patients and communities alike. PMS does, however, possess some unique attributes to enable more responsive services. It enhances the autonomy of primary care professionals while at the same time increasing their accountability, which is apt as quality and accountability are increasingly two of the most important aims of any health care system the world over.

PMS reinforces the point that the primary health care team, not individual professionals, working to a registered list of patients is the building block of health care in the UK. PMS offers the opportunity to reduce unnecessary bureaucracy and to reward outcomes of care, not simply process. It encourages workforce flexibility and skill mix, and is of great value in recruitment and retention, preserving all that is good about UK primary care yet ensuring increasing professionalisation where it is needed, e.g. in human resource management and practice organisation. It complements the role of primary care groups and primary care trusts as it is a vehicle for a two-way contractual relationship, it begins to significantly address the under-provision of services in socially deprived areas, and it encourages a public health focus.

As this book demonstrates, the evidence is partial and we may never be able to assess the impact of PMS in terms of health outcomes. PMS is not the only way forward, but it is nevertheless changing the face of primary care.

David Colin-Thomé
National Clinical Director for Primary Care, Associate Director London Regional Office of the Department of Health and GP at Castlefields Health Centre, Runcorn, Cheshire

Introduction

Richard Lewis and Stephen Gillam

In April 1998, when the first personal medical services (PMS) pilots went live, it was far from clear that this new policy signalled a radical departure for primary care in England. Indeed, it seemed possible that the early pilots would wither and the scheme would silently slip from view. The collective focus of the NHS was firmly on the rising stars of primary care groups (PCGs) and primary care trusts (PCTs). When we published our first report on PMS pilots in 1999,[1] the significance of these pilots was just becoming apparent: a second wave was just getting under way and Ministers were taking notice of a phenomenon that was growing largely of its own accord.

In 2001, some two years later, things look rather different. The NHS Plan has confirmed the long-term place of PMS within a 'modern' NHS (before, it should be noted, the formal outputs of the national evaluation had been received). Recruitment to the scheme has soared, with more than 20 per cent of GPs and 24 per cent of the population within the scheme by the third wave, and a fourth wave on the horizon (see Table I.1 below). At the same time, the future of general medical services

Table I.1 Numbers of 'live' PMS pilots

NHSE Region	Live pilots Wave 1	Live pilots Wave 2	Live pilots Wave 3	Live pilots All Waves
North Yorkshire	14	18	134	166
Eastern	7	18	46	71
Trent	9	10	58	77
South Eastern	9	27	98	134
London	12	53	193	258
North West	13	23	51	87
West Midlands	13	15	108	136
South Western	7	21	84	112
Total	**84**	**185**	**772**	**1041**

Source: Department of Health

(GMS) looks in doubt. Labelled as 'inadequate' by both government and the profession, it is not clear what the alternative to PMS will look like (indeed, as we argue later in this book, GMS and PMS seem set on a path of convergence).

It is worth remembering that PMS pilots (and personal dental pilots) have their roots in the 'listening exercise' of 1996 carried out by Gerald Malone, then Conservative Minister for Health. This is important, not just because it demonstrates a shared policy vision that transcends party allegiances, but because PMS pilots were designed to solve the numerous (and entrenched) problems that had been identified by front-line professionals and managers. The stakes, therefore, were high. The guidance accompanying the first wave of pilots underlined the Government's expectations of PMS. Pilots were to deliver primary care with improved fairness, efficiency, effectiveness, responsiveness, integration, flexibility and accountability.[2] A tall order, indeed.

What are PMS pilots?

PMS pilots are diverse and difficult to categorise – indeed, that is the point of them. They are locally designed services tailored to meet the needs of local populations. Yet they all share a number of important characteristics:

- PMS pilots are governed by a local contract negotiated between a provider and the commissioner (either a health authority or a PCT). Under GMS, primary care providers are bound by the national contract for GPs negotiated between the Department of Health and the General Practice Committee of the British Medical Association. Since the third wave of PMS in 2001, all pilots must comply with a 'national contractual framework' that sets out the basic structure of the contract, while leaving scope for local discretion.
- PMS pilots are based on a local cash limit that sets out the resource assumptions for the pilot in advance of its operation. This contrasts with GMS, where a significant proportion of contract resources are 'non-cash-limited'. Under GMS, resources for any individual GP are determined retrospectively and will depend greatly on the levels of activity carried out in-year. There is, however, a national cash limit that is applied to GPs collectively.

• PMS pilots are open to a wide range of providers, including NHS trusts, PCTs, other NHS professionals (for example nurses) and, in exceptional circumstances, limited companies as long as these are owned by 'members of the NHS family'. The national GMS contract is available only to appropriately qualified GPs who are accepted onto a health authority medical list.

PMS pilots are often associated with the rise of the salaried GP. Indeed, opponents of the scheme suggest that PMS is simply a vehicle for ensuring that all GPs become salaried. In fact, the association between PMS pilots and salaried practice is significant but not causal. Salaried practice is certainly an option under PMS but is by no means compulsory – the vast majority of PMS GPs have remained independent contractors.

PMS pilots can take one of two basic contractual types (see Box I.1).

Box I.1 'PMS' OR 'PMS PLUS'?

• **PMS pilots** provide the broad range of GMS services a patient would expect to receive from any GP, but cash limited and operating within a locally specified and negotiated contract.

• **PMS Plus pilots** extend the range of services by including non-GMS services such as community nursing or specialist services such as extended disease management, sexual health or services for refugees. This type of pilot has a single contract combining hospital and community health services (HCHS) and GMS funding, but does not have a purchasing role.

Significantly, 'PMS Plus' has allowed providers to continue to deliver a range of additional services from within primary care, notwithstanding the abolition of GP fundholding. Indeed, PMS Plus simplifies this process and removes many of the conflicts of interest in the merging of purchasing and providing roles inherent in GP fundholding. Perhaps curiously, 'PMS Plus' has been little used and, in the third wave, applications have been received with only tepid enthusiasm in some areas.

Has PMS delivered?

The expectations of PMS have been such that, barring a miracle, they could scarcely be fully met. Yet PMS has risen to some of the challenges set out for it. Evaluation, both our own at the King's Fund and that of the national evaluation team,[3,4,5] has begun to demonstrate ways in which PMS pilots are delivering improvements in patient care. In general, pilots:

- are creating new roles for professionals
- are targeting deprived or needy populations
- have increased quality of care against a number of indicators
- have successfully recruited scarce medical staff.

However, the extent to which these improvements can wholly be laid at the door of PMS is a different question. As we have already observed, PMS pilots did not develop in isolation. PCG/Ts, clinical governance and the NHS Plan are just three initiatives that have developed in parallel. Labour's 'modernisation' of the NHS has altered primary care in many different ways and each strand of this modernisation has impacted on and been affected by the other. The PMS experiment has slipped the confines of its petri dish and is busy consorting with other experiments in the NHS laboratory. We cannot be sure that the evaluation of PMS has not been contaminated.

About this book

This book is designed to give the reader information about the early years of the PMS phenomenon. It assumes a level of knowledge about the 'nuts and bolts' of the PMS pilot process and is not intended to be a source of detailed information on the mechanics of the piloting process, still less a 'how to' guide for aspirant pilots. Instead, our focus has been on the myriad ways in which pilots have sought to use PMS pilots to achieve local aims. This book also charts the progress of a small number of pilots in more detail.

The book is split into three sections:

Section one: a report on an independent evaluation of PMS pilots

Here we present the findings of two evaluations carried out by the King's Fund. First, Clare Jenkins reports on case studies of four first wave pilots in London. She describes the diverse experiences of the sites, reflecting on their successes and limitations. This offers an interesting comparison between the 'practice-led' and the 'trust-led' pilots – in terms of their focus, management and outcomes. Second, Richard Lewis presents summary findings of an evaluation of the nine first wave 'nurse-led' PMS pilots. These pilots are among the most radical experiments set in train by PMS. Here nurses, rather than doctors, provide leadership within the primary health care team and significantly increase their clinical roles.

Section two: reflections on pilots in progress

We have brought together a number of short commentaries about the practical application of PMS pilots from those directly involved in leading pilots or commissioning them. These are not intended to be representative; indeed, they have been selected because in many respects they reflect the greatest level of innovation and have tackled issues that we believe will be of significant strategic importance to primary care in the future. Nor should these short chapters be seen as independent evaluations; that is not their purpose. Instead, they are impressionistic and designed to give a flavour of what has, for some, been an intense process. We have encouraged the authors to share their personal experiences and some have 'shot from the hip'.

Tim Crossley reports on a scheme in Wolverhampton that offers structured salaried employment to GPs. A new Directorate of Primary Care within the community NHS trust has 'converted' a number of single-handed independent contractor GPs as well as establishing new salaried practices in areas of high need. This is a model that PCTs should find useful as they become more active in shaping local primary care services.

James Kingsland describes his pilot's attempts to develop practice-based services and to reclaim clinical work currently (and in his view, unnecessarily) carried out in hospital. By persuading his health authority to fund new primary care services, his practice dramatically reduced its reliance on hospital care – and broke even!

Catherine Baraniak and Lance Gardner, two independent contractor nurses providing 'nurse-led' services, describe their unique brand of PMS pilot. These have inverted the traditional hierarchy within primary care, in terms of both the power and the clinical relationships within the primary care team. In these pilots, nurses provide much of the first contact care and the formal leadership of the team. Catherine and Lance have been seen as pioneers of nurse-led care and have attracted much attention within the nursing profession as well as some controversy from outside it.

Tim Richardson and Andrew Roscoe describe the Integrated Care Partnership in Epsom, Surrey. This is a large primary care organisation that brought together three independent practices. The Partnership provides one of the largest PMS Plus pilots. A full range of specialist care (including that of consultants) is provided as part of a primary care-led service that is truly challenging the traditional primary–secondary care divide.

In contrast, Rigo Pizarro-Duhart provides the commissioner's experience. The history of the first two waves of PMS has very much been one of individual pilots developing in splendid isolation – but not in south-east London. There, the early take-up of PMS pilots was exceptional, with 30 per cent of the health authority population covered by first and second wave pilots (increasing to more than 70 per cent in wave three). This has proved challenging for the health authority, which had to develop its capacity quickly. Rigo outlines some of these challenges, as well as the techniques and mechanisms put in place to cope with them. Again, with the take-up of the third wave on a sharply upward curve (which, it seems safe to assume, will continue with future waves), these experiences should prove valuable to health authorities and PCTs.

Section three: conclusions – PMS pilots and the 'modernisation' of primary care

Here we consider the PMS phenomenon so far. Drawing on our own and other evaluations, as well as the experiences of our 'leading edge' contributors, we examine the strengths and weaknesses of PMS pilots in relation to the governmental agenda for primary care. What is meant by

NHS 'modernisation', and has PMS demonstrated that it can be the vehicle for change that the Government hoped for? What will be its impact on government–professional relations, and how will PMS change the shape and delivery of primary care services on the ground?

References

1 Lewis R, Gillam S, editors. *Transforming primary care – personal medical services in the new NHS*. London: King's Fund, 1999.
2 Department of Health. *Personal medical services under the NHS (Primary Care) Act 1997: a comprehensive guide*. London: NHS Executive, 1997.
3 National Primary Care Research and Development Centre. *National evaluation of first wave NHS personal medical services pilots: integrated interim report from four research projects*. Manchester: NPCRDC, 2000.
4 Lewis R, Gillam S, editors. *Transforming primary care – personal medical services in the new NHS*. London: King's Fund, 1999.
5 Lewis R. *Nurse-led primary care: learning from PMS pilots*. London: King's Fund, 2001.

Section one

Chapter 1

Learning from four London PMS pilots – report on the King's Fund evaluation of first wave PMS pilots

Clare Jenkins

Introduction

The King's Fund has recently completed a three-year local evaluation of four of the original 12 first wave London PMS pilots. The pilot sites were chosen to reflect the range of sites nationally, and included two practice-based and two trust-led pilots, one of which was nurse-led.

Our evaluation was a multi-method case study of four very different pilot sites (described in Boxes 1.1 to 1.4), each with its own specific objectives and often with very different registered populations. We adapted our methodology to each of the sites (see Table 1.1), allowing the pilots to 'tell their own stories' through wide-ranging interviews with key stakeholders. In addition to in-depth interviews, further data collection methods included:

- focus groups with individuals and organisations working closely with particular client groups identified as a priority by the pilots
- a patient satisfaction questionnaire (the General Practice Assessment Survey* – GPAS[1])
- a practice profile questionnaire
- an audit of chronic disease management.

An analysis of the cost-effectiveness of the pilots was not within the remit of our study. With the exception of the interview schedules and the

* GPAS is copyright of Safran/The Health Institute and National Primary Care Research and Development Centre.

Table 1.1 Case studies and evaluation methods

	North Hillingdon	SW London	Isleworth	Lambeth
No. of practices	3	7	1	1
Practice characteristics	PMS Practice-based Salaried GP option	PMS Plus Practice-based	PMS Plus Trust-led Salaried GPs	PMS Trust-led Nurse-led Salaried GPs
Annual interviews	n=29	n=65	n=31	n=29
Angina audit*	Mar 2000 n=41	Mar 2000 n=103	Dec 2000 n=3	Dec 2000 n=0
GPAS*	1: Sep 1999 2: Sep 2000 n=694 (58%)	1: Nov 1998 2: Sep 2000 n=1562 (56%)	Sep 2000 n=95 (48%)	Sep 2000 n=22 (11%)
Practice profile questionnaire*	1: Apr 1999 2: Dec 2000	1: Nov 1998 2: Dec 2000	1: Feb 1999 2: Dec 2000	1: Apr 1999 2: Dec 2000
Focus group	Not applicable	Sep 2000	Mar 2000	Apr 2000
Registration questionnaire	Not applicable	Not applicable	Spring 1999	Not applicable

* also used in the national evaluation

focus groups, the research tools replicated the data collection methods used in the National Primary Care Research and Development Centre national evaluation. This allows data collected in our evaluation to be compared with a larger sample of PMS pilots and a control group of GMS pilots across the country.

The data collected during this evaluation were presented in four case study reports, supplemented by feedback and discussion meetings arranged with each of the sites.[2,3,4,5] This chapter provides a summary of the findings from these case studies and draws out issues that might have relevance to other PMS pilots. Of course, there are difficulties in generalising from case studies. Where there are particular qualifications that should be taken into account, we set these out.

A number of major themes arose from the various methods of data collection:

- local contracting
- quality of care

- accessibility
- partnership working
- relationship with other organisations
- roles
- workload
- trust-led primary care.

We address each of these in turn in this chapter.

Local contracting

One of the key differences between PMS pilots and their GMS counterparts was the opportunity delivered by the new legislation for PMS pilots to negotiate their contracts locally, giving them more flexibility to cater for the particular needs of their local populations. Content analysis of the early PMS pilot contracts suggested that they were 'surprisingly limited'[6] and, in the first year at least, did not differ greatly from the national contract (colloquially known as the 'Red Book'):

> ... what we didn't want to do was to write a contract from scratch in haste, which then set a precedent which we were locked into. We went for a very fluid level of contracting and we'll negotiate different parts later. 'Red Book nouveau' we call it ...
>
> (health authority, year 1)

The workload that resulted from negotiating the contracts was onerous, and PMS pilot and health authority staff reported that they had been surprised by both the depth and the level of work involved in moving to a new method of contracting.

Contracts were not always easy to negotiate – being described as 'tortuous and tedious', and 'painful' in some cases – which may have influenced the less-than-positive relationships some pilots reported with their health authority. For their part, health authority staff felt that negotiating in such a 'highly risky area with profound national consequences' did not sit happily with the timescales and levels of staffing, and they described the experience as being like 'navigating in an unfamiliar world with piranhas nearby'. Significantly, three of the four pilots made no changes to the formal contract over the lifetime of the pilots.

The pilots often felt that they were not sufficiently supported by their health authorities, a point of view that the health authorities themselves agreed with. First wave PMS pilots were set up at a time of huge organisational change, and the health authorities reported that they had both underestimated the level of involvement needed and, at the same time, had 'bigger fish to fry' – with PCG boundaries to be negotiated and, later, with the setting up of the first PCTs. There was a view that, had the pilots featured more highly in health authorities' lists of priorities, they may well have made more progress.

A significant concern, and one that may have increasing resonance as the Government encourages the move to PMS, was expressed by the health authorities. They felt that the need to monitor individually the quality of PMS pilots had made, and would continue to make, a much greater demand on them than was the case with GMS practices.

Both the crowded political agenda and the heavy workloads involved were seen as having had an adverse impact on the health authorities' ability to engage fully with the first wave PMS pilots. However, the early contracts, although rudimentary, were seen as being a solid basis on which to develop something more sophisticated for the future.

Quality of care

The four pilots involved in our evaluation set out with different aims and objectives; consequently, we adopted a multi-method approach to assess the different dimensions of quality the pilots aimed to address. All four pilots perceived that they were providing high-quality primary care, and we used three quality indicators to review more objectively the practices' self-reported views:

- a survey of patients' views (GPAS)
- an audit of chronic disease management in relation to angina
- a practice profile questionnaire.

The GPAS was sent to 200 randomly selected patients, aged 16 and over, who had been registered at one of the 12 practices for more than a year. The GPAS was designed to assess those aspects of care most valued by patients in nine sub-scales:

- access
- interpersonal care
- receptionists
- trust
- continuity of care
- doctor's knowledge of the patient
- technical care
- practice nursing care
- communication.

The questionnaire was used twice in the practice-based pilots, but only once in the trust-led pilots as, being new practices, their patients had not been registered for the required length of time when the first questionnaire was sent out.

For the practice pilots, there was a very small degree of variability in results between the first and second round of GPAS. While there was no improvement in patients' perceptions of quality over the lifetime of the pilots, this could be because the timescale was simply too short for patients to discern changes in quality (rather than reflecting a failure of PMS). This latter view was implied by one of the health authorities:

> To date, from the perception of the patients, I would say that the advantages to them are not that visible – they would largely be behind the scenes.
>
> (health authority, year 2)

The results for the later round of GPAS for all participating pilots are given in Figure 1.1 below. It is striking that trust-led pilots generally scored less highly than the practice-based pilots. Scores were lower, in particular, on the 'continuity' and 'knowledge of patient' scales. There are likely to be a number of reasons for these observed differences.

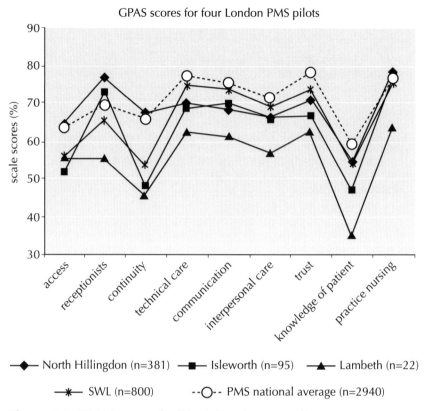

Figure 1.1 GPAS* scores for King's Fund case studies

For new practices, it is perhaps not surprising that 'knowledge of patient' scores are relatively low and the impact of significant staff turnover at both trust sites is likely to have been reflected in the 'continuity' scores. However, it is disappointing that practices specifically set up to improve accessibility have not scored more highly on the 'access' scale.

Inter-practice variability is also striking (see Figure 1.2 below, which shows scale scores for two practices in one of the practice-based pilots). This demonstrates that multi-practice pilots should not be treated as homogeneous organisations. Patients clearly perceive the quality of the service they receive very differently within the constituent practices. This should provide useful learning within pilots as they attempt to universalise best practice.

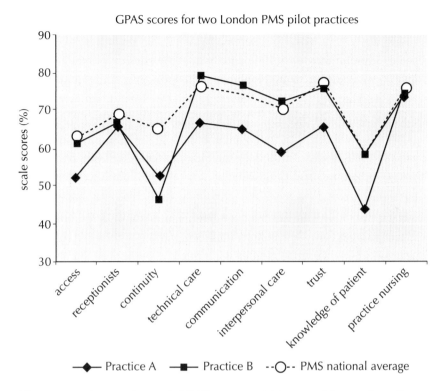

GPAS scores for two London PMS pilot practices

—◆— Practice A　—■— Practice B　--○-- PMS national average

Figure 1.2 Comparison of GPAS scores within a multi-practice pilot

However, when making inter-practice and inter-pilot comparisons it is worth bearing several factors in mind. Response rates to patient satisfaction questionnaires may be lower in London.[7] For one of the participating pilots, the response was 11 per cent – making meaningful comparisons between the practices problematic. Whether practices are doing 'relatively well' or 'badly' may be related to a range of population and/or environmental factors that have not been analysed. Satisfaction surveys typically yield little variability in results, with certain groups of patients, particularly older patients, tending to express greater levels of satisfaction with the services they receive. The two trust-led pilots, in particular, recorded younger mean ages for GPAS respondents than the two practice-based pilots.

When compared with the national evaluation PMS pilot practices (and non-PMS controls), the four London PMS pilots generally showed lower (some much lower) scores. Although the national evaluation pilots were chosen to demonstrate a mix of demographic and organisational features and include pilots in deprived areas, none of the pilot practices were located in London or the south-east. It is possible that there may be, as in the level of response to questionnaires, a 'London effect' in the way that patients rate the quality of services they receive (also a finding of the national patient survey[7]).

We next looked at chronic disease management as a measure of clinical quality. The Angina Audit, used in the national evaluation in five PMS pilot practices and five matched non-PMS controls, was designed to evaluate the clinical care and note-taking for patients with angina. In replicating the use of this questionnaire, the King's Fund evaluation analysed data from 11 of the 12 participating practices. Patients receiving a repeat prescription for a 'top 20' angina drug in the six months prior to the questionnaire being completed were eligible for inclusion. Up to 20 patients were selected randomly from each practice. Several of the practices were unable to identify 20 patients and one practice failed to identify any patients who fulfilled the inclusion criteria (this was not unreasonable given the size and demographic structure of the practice's list).

Overall, angina audit scores were higher in the three participating London PMS pilots than in the PMS comparator practices and non-PMS controls (see Table 1.2). While this is an encouraging result for the pilots themselves, our results present a snapshot of quality at one point in time and are not necessarily evidence of quality improvement directly attributable to PMS pilot status. The results are also likely to have been influenced by the differing methodologies used by the national evaluation and the King's Fund evaluation teams – the national evaluation questionnaires were completed by a team of researchers whereas the practices taking part in the King's Fund evaluation

Table 1.2 Audit of angina care

Site	Mean score	Number	Standard deviation
Isleworth	65.00	3	8.66
SW London	65.80	103	21.49
North Hillingdon	72.65	38	19.04
National PMS	55.60	78	18.26
National non-PMS controls	62.50	100	25.14

completed their own questionnaires. However, the results do appear to suggest that the practice-based pilots are providing high-quality care in this aspect of service delivery, and that the new trust-led pilot was able to score as highly as more well-established practices (although the numbers of observations was extremely small).

The practice profile questionnaire was the third questionnaire used to assess pilot quality that replicated the national evaluation study. The questionnaire was based on Health Authority Performance Indicators (HAPI) against which quality of care can be assessed,[8] and all the indicators have been validated[9] for the following areas:

- access and availability
- range of services provided
- care for chronic conditions
- prescribing.

The data collected described a range of practice characteristics (for example, whether the practice was registered for child health surveillance, minor surgery and maternity care, and whether patients can get an urgent appointment on the same day). The questionnaire was sent out to the four London PMS pilot sites between November 1998 and April 1999, and again in December 2000 to provide a 'before and after' picture of the practices' development during their first three years of PMS status. Again, the data from the King's Fund evaluation have been compared with data from the national evaluation PMS pilot sites and non-PMS control sites (shown in Table 1.3).

Scores on the practice profile questionnaire were high, and 100 per cent in many cases (though it was designed so that practices *could* score highly).[10] Some apparent changes in the range of services provided may reflect differences in recording between the two data collection points, rather than real changes in quality. Although useful descriptive data are generated, this may not be a particularly discriminating tool.

Accessibility

Issues of accessibility included physical access to the practices (for example, opening hours and location as measured from the patients'

Table 1.3 Audit of angina chronic disease management

	Number of participating practices Year		Organisation score (%) Year		Access score (%) Year		Prescribing score (%) Year		Chronic disease management score (%) Year	
	1	2	1	2	1	2	1	2	1	2
Isleworth	1	1	67	100	75	100	40	80	64	82
North Hillingdon	3	3	89	100	75	83	73	87	85	100
Lambeth	1	1	33	0	75	100	80	80	73	64
SW London	6	5	100	100	96	85	90	88	86	93
PMS national evaluation	23	23	94	96	80	84	68	75	72	86

perspective, using GPAS), as well as access to services for marginalised groups of patients who had traditionally found it difficult to register with mainstream general practice. Clearly, access was a key priority for the trust-led sites that had been set up in areas where problems had been identified for patients seeking to register. Both trust pilots felt that they had been successful in attracting the target groups they had specifically set out to reach, and described the mix of patients sitting in the waiting room as being 'totally different' from that of neighbouring practices:

I often feel that we have a lot more of the kinds of patients that other practices would shut their lists to. That's good, because that's what we were set up for, but it's very hard work. I often feel that our patients aren't very 'well trained' if you know what I mean – they don't understand the processes, or how the NHS works. They ask all sorts of non-general practice questions, which I'm sure most GMS practices wouldn't get.

(trust-led pilot, year 3)

Patients were described as being 'high demand', often with multiple problems and, in many cases, requiring the services of a translator. In addition, the 'newness' of the patients to the practice (at the time of interview, all the patients had been registered for less than two years) meant that they were generally not well known to the clinicians, requiring more background work. This, together with the rapid list growth, meant that the practices experienced difficulties in expanding their lists smoothly and managing the take-on of patients. As a result, policies were adopted to manage patient registration (for example, refusing registration to patients already registered with a local GP).

The practices' own perceptions that they had been successful in providing greater access to particular groups of patients were confirmed by the focus group meetings held at both the trust-led pilots. Often, this was the result of immense flexibility on the part of the pilots – in particular, providing instant access on demand if this was appropriate (for example, where new refugees might be 'lost' to the NHS if not seen immediately). Conversely, attendees at the focus groups graphically described the difficulty they had in registering their patients in 'mainstream' practices in the area, and the frustration of sending their clients to A&E departments when they failed to register them at local general practices.

While the outcomes of the focus groups were generally very positive, intention and enthusiasm have not always matched the reality of improving access. In one of the practices in particular, the rapid turnover of reception staff meant that protocols concerning the registration of new patients were not always followed, making registration at the practice difficult at times. This underlines the need for effective local management to support the overall 'mission' of the pilots.

Respondents to the patient satisfaction questionnaire in one of the trust-led pilots reported that they had to wait a long time for their appointments to start (22 per cent waited for 45 minutes or more), almost a quarter (23 per cent) had to wait four or more days to gain an appointment with any GP, yet they were satisfied with the length of time the doctor spent with them:

> ... [the patients] feel the GPs have got the time to sit and listen. That's what the patients say to me ... In other surgeries, they've got their five-minute slot, its 'Oh, take these painkillers, we'll send you up to the specialist', without getting at what the basic problem is.
>
> (trust-led pilot, year 2)

Local evaluation work carried out in this pilot suggested that appointment lengths were long – often very long.[11] There is a difficult balance to be met between length of consultations and access. While patients may have been critical of certain aspects of access, both the trust-led practices offer open-access sessions in their practices.

Overall, the practices felt certain that they were meeting unmet need and, by the end of year one, both practices had registered over 1000 patients – a rapid take-on of patients by any standard.

Partnership working

Staff in all four pilots were extremely enthusiastic about the potential they felt that PMS offered them for closer working relations with other organisations. For the practice-based pilots, closer links with the other practices making up the PMS pilots were valued as a means of gaining experience from observing the clinical practice of their pilot colleagues:

> Being single-handed, I was on my own. Now I've got the benefit of a group, while maintaining my independence – I get the benefits of both.
>
> (practice-based pilot, year 2)

For the trust-led pilots, there was enthusiasm to work more collaboratively from both pilot staff and staff in organisations working closely with the pilots' identified client groups. Particular successes included the closer working relationships that had been built up with drug users' organisations and refugee workers in the Lambeth pilot, and with voluntary organisations in the Isleworth pilot:

> Now that the NSPCC [is co-located], we put together a package where children can go to a playgroup for a couple of sessions a week and the local social services fund it – a very inexpensive but amazingly effective package.
>
> (trust-led pilot, year 2)

For one of the trust-led pilots in particular, the local authority had been heavily involved in the establishment of the pilot, giving valuable commitment and support to the project.

However, pilots were also aware of potential links that had not been made, and there was some sense of disappointment that opportunities had been missed to work even more collaboratively, a finding consistent with the national evaluation.[12] In the practice-based pilots, even where staff had seen the benefits of liaising with colleagues in other practices, the reality was that collaborative meetings were not always well attended.

Relationship with other organisations

PMS and local general practice

Relations between PMS pilots and other local primary care services were often difficult. There was clear hostility from some local doctors, particularly directed at the trust-led pilots. In seeking to register new patients, they were seen as a threat to the viability of neighbouring practices. However, while neighbouring practices might be concerned that the new pilots could end up 'nicking' their patients, the pilots themselves felt that more demanding or geographically outlying patients from local practices were being directed towards them. Anecdotal evidence to this effect was obtained from a number of sources.

This raises an important question about access. Are the new practices that target marginalised populations, such as the two evaluated here, genuinely increasing access or simply serving to realign the provision of care? Will PMS create 'ghetto' practices serving populations such as the homeless or refugees, albeit providing them with high-quality services?

Common to all four pilots were the negative responses generated by Local Medical Committees (LMCs). While the LMCs stated that they were not anti-PMS pilots *per se*, several expressed a 'not in my backyard' attitude towards the existence of first wave PMS pilots in their local areas, viewing the pilots as being preferentially funded and disadvantaging GMS practices.

> I think [PMS pilots] have to be shown to offer something that traditional general practice finds it difficult to target, for example homeless [people], drug users. It's daft as a replacement for ordinary general practice.
>
> (LMC, year 2)

PMS, PCGs and health authorities

A degree of isolation of the PMS pilots within their respective PCGs was reported:

> We're still a bit of an anomaly. Other practices in the PCG are still wary of us. I get the impression that they think we shouldn't really be here – due to the misunderstanding that the health authority are throwing money at us. They think we're on a cushy number.
>
> (trust-led pilot, year 2)

While there was some suggestion that the PMS pilots had not 'joined in' with the activities of their PCG as much as other practices had (an 'us and them' situation), there was also a sense that the PCGs had not been fully involved with the PMS pilots. First wave pilots had often sprung up prior to PCGs becoming fully operational. In this sense, they were not the PCGs' 'babies'.

The health authorities, as described earlier, expressed regret that they had not engaged fully with the PMS pilots from the beginning. The pilots felt that, as part of a groundbreaking first wave, they were having to 'sell' the PMS initiative to the health authorities and persuade them that it was worth supporting. Some pilots, too, looked for more support than the health authorities felt able to give, while others needed less support as the pilots became more established. As successive waves of pilots were launched, raising PMS up the political agenda, the health authorities became more supportive, at least in principle. Overall, good relationships between the health authorities and the PMS pilots were maintained or improved over time:

> It's certainly been a relationship that's had its ups and downs. At the moment [it's] quite good, and better than it was before the pilot, but there have been times when it was a lot worse.
>
> (health authority, year 2)

The role of health authorities, at least for later waves, will be less crucial as responsibility for pilots passes to PCTs.

Roles

One of the key aims of the PMS pilot initiative nationally was to 'provide opportunities and incentives for primary care professionals to use their skills to the full'.[13] Later on, the Government specifically called for pilots that offered other professionals, particularly nurses, 'the opportunity to be full partners and explore the better use of skill mix'.[14] All four pilots had appointed new staff, including a mental health advisor in South West London and a nurse practitioner in North Hillingdon. All posts in the trust-led pilots were new posts. The practice-based pilots stated that they were making better use of skill mix. However, our evaluation did not collect data on staffing levels, so we were unable to confirm this:

> [The pilot is] beginning now to use flexibilities of PMS, to look at different ways of meeting requirements. It isn't an automatic 'Let's put another partner in'. So they're looking at 'Should we use salaried assistants?', 'Should we use nurse practitioners?'.
>
> (practice-led pilot, year 3)

However, PMS appeared to make little difference to GP roles. The GPs we interviewed did not feel that their clinical roles had changed (apart from the pilot leads who had taken on extra work in setting up the pilots). The national evaluation has described the development of nursing roles in PMS pilots.[15] In our evaluation, nurses felt that they were carrying out new work (for example, triage and additional clinics); however, they did not attribute this directly to PMS:

> My job hasn't changed at all since last [interview]. There are areas I've moved into in care – but not because of PMS pilots ...
>
> (practice-led pilot, year 2)

Administrative staff felt that pilot status had impacted on their roles, for example in giving 'guided tours' around the practice to those interested in moving to PMS status, and in giving presentations. However, this work related to their status as a PMS pilot, rather than to the aspirations of the pilot. While a reduction in bureaucracy was a much-heralded benefit of PMS, some practice managers found themselves collecting more data and answering more requests for information than they had previously.

At the extreme, the nurse-led pilot sought to implement a very different model of primary care. This proved problematic. It was planned that the nurse would take on a leading clinical and management role in the practice and that, in addition, reception staff would be multi-skilled to carry out tasks such as taking blood specimens. In practice, it proved extremely difficult to conceptualise or operationalise these roles:

> *In terms of nurse-led – we change that every day! We're not winning on that.*
>
> (trust-led pilot, year 3)

> *Patients generally need to know the boundaries of the person they're going to see – if they're used to seeing [receptionists] stood behind a desk answering the phone, they're going to be a bit perturbed when they ask them to roll up their sleeve and take some blood, because that's not how it is.*
>
> (trust-led pilot, year 2)

First wave nurse-led pilots, albeit small in number, have pushed back boundaries in developing pioneering roles for nurses (as discussed in Chapters 2 and 5 [16,17]) However, this has not been without difficulties, as the high turnover of staff testifies.

It is not surprising that pre-existing roles within PMS pilots have changed little. The practice-based pilots in particular are still heavily associated with the lead GPs who initiated the projects, and far less with other members of staff:

> *Mere mortals like me don't get involved.*
>
> (practice-based pilot, year 2)

Interview data collected over successive years suggested that, though the levels of engagement of other practice staff increased as the pilots progressed, the view that 'people like me just want to do their job' was not uncommon:

I hate [the political] side of it – the organisational, PCG, PMS, whatever ... I'm just not particularly interested in it, and that's the bit that I find drags me down really.

(practice-based pilot, year 2)

PMS is highly associated with salaried practice, and this was a significant feature of our case studies. One of the practice-based pilots, in addition to the two trust-led pilots, had appointed salaried GPs. However, salaried roles introduced some difficult tensions. Several of the salaried GPs we spoke to reported a difficult balance between having full clinical responsibility on the one hand, while not being able to make decisions about the running of the practice on the other:

I'm not the boss. I'm being told what to do. On an irritable day, I'm quite annoyed that I don't have full responsibility – though I do clinically, so I would like the whole responsibility at times.

(trust-led pilot, year 2)

One of the trusts took a rather different view. It felt that, as a trust running a general practice, it *would* expect to manage the pilot. While this meant that the GPs have less autonomy than they would have experienced under GMS, this may be an inevitable and natural consequence of trust-led primary care. Any desire on the part of a salaried GP to enjoy full autonomy and control, while divesting himself/herself of managerial responsibilities, might be seen as unrealistic and misplaced. Nevertheless, in this particular trust, discussions were underway with the practice to consider whether greater responsibility might be delegated in the future, given the increasing maturity of the pilot.

In debating the merits or otherwise of salaried status, several of the salaried GPs we spoke to said that, when looking for their next job, they would be likely to move out of PMS and into a traditional GMS partnership (and, indeed, some did so). Others said that they would actively seek to work in another PMS pilot. As intended, salaried general practice within a PMS pilot appears to offer greater choice to doctors and the opportunity to plan a career:

> *... there are various stages in your life when PMS is a good place to be, and there are stages in your life when it isn't – and some people will like it and some people won't ...*
>
> (trust-led pilot, year 3)

Conversely, while the pilots' salaried posts were felt to have encouraged high-quality staff into an area, the downside of salaried status was the high turnover of staff. This caused upheaval and insecurity, and compromised the longitudinal qualities of primary care.

Workload

A reduction in the bureaucracy associated with the GMS contract was anticipated by PMS pilot staff in the first round of interviews. However, all four practices continued to record the Item of Service payments upon which part of the GMS contract was based. Ultimately, there was little evidence that, in the short term at least, PMS had delivered a significant reduction in administration. Indeed, the development of the pilots carried an administrative burden.

The issue of clinical workload becomes a significant issue in trust-led pilots. Inevitably, new practices enjoyed a high clinical capacity while lists remained low. At the outset, staff felt that they could offer long consultations and meet the needs of a deprived population in accord with their ambitious proposals; this contrasted with the experience of GMS practice. However, as list sizes grew, staff reported significantly increased work pressure and were unable to maintain the level of service. They became concerned about the impact this might have on the quality of services they offered:

> *... at the beginning we had time, you know, if it took an hour for an appointment with the interpreters – to ring everybody round, to sort everything out – we could do it, whereas we can't do it anymore.*
>
> (trust-led pilot, year 2)

There was also concern that, in struggling to cope with 'the sheer weight of patients', the practice would begin to lose its focus on marginalised groups. PMS pilots received no preferential funding for the day-to-day running of their practices; indeed, the level of resources provided to these pilots was keenly monitored by other local general practices. A clear mismatch emerged between the expectations of the pilots that they would be able to work in new and innovative ways and the reality of moving towards average list sizes and having only enough time to 'just see patients'.

Staff in the trust-led pilots felt that they were registering a 'different kind of patient', and that the 'newness' of the patients, their high levels of need and their mobility caused high levels of workload:

> *It's a very demanding practice – our patients need time.*
>
> (trust-led pilot, year 2)

In addition, the high mobility of patients (some of whom move into local hostels for a short time, move away, and perhaps return some months later) led staff to describe their work as 'disjointed':

> *… you put in an enormous amount of effort, and three weeks later they've gone … There aren't the 'highs', the relationships you get with a normal caseload.*
>
> (trust-led pilot, year 2)

Despite the heavy workloads, staff in trust-led pilots felt that they faced a level of scepticism from their GP colleagues. At one of the pilots, a PCG representative commented that 'if you're a one man practice, then you should be able to do one man's work', while PMS pilot staff felt that they were constantly being checked up on to see how large their list size was:

> *… doctors say '1200 [registered patients]! You wimps, we've got 3000!'.*
>
> (trust-led pilot, year 2)

The response of pilot staff was an emphatic 'I can justify my workload to anybody', and this raises the important question of whether staff–patient ratios need to be different in practices specifically set up to register high-need patients.

Trust-led primary care

The involvement of NHS trusts in the provision of PMS introduced new dynamics into an environment hitherto characterised by the predominance of small organisations. The input of information technology and finance departments of the community trusts was recognised as being valuable in the setting up of the two trust-led PMS pilots. In addition, the financial benefits of trusts setting up new primary care services should not be underestimated. Evaluative work carried out independently by one of the trust-led pilots suggested that, had the pilot been set up as a GMS practice, it would have made a significant financial loss, at least in the early years.[18]

Members of trust management who had initiated the pilots were also extremely enthusiastic about the potential their pilots would offer in areas where primary care services were under pressure. Co-locating a number of different services, not always those found in more traditional general practices, was seen as being very positive, and expectations of what the new services could deliver were high.

However, staff in the practices themselves reported that they found it difficult to work under the operational umbrella of a larger organisation. Decision-makers were not always based on site, leading to a feeling of having to check 'with a million people first' before decisions were made, coupled with a slow response time and a lack of autonomy that staff found frustrating:

> *The big organisation doesn't understand the small organisation's needs.*
>
> (trust-led pilot, year 2)

When describing the operational difficulties of running a general practice under the umbrella of a larger organisation, the new model of working was often compared unfavourably to the more traditional GMS by the staff we interviewed:

> *In GMS practices, you'd ask the senior partner – the difference is that it's somebody within the practice – someone outside can't always appreciate the significance.*
>
> (trust-led pilot, year 2)

In both the practice-based and the trust-led pilots there was questioning of how different PMS really was from traditional GMS practices, with a common feeling that, workwise, it was 'the same as before':

> *From a patient sense, I can't think of any difference at all. There have been remarkably few changes between this and GMS, actually.*
>
> (trust-led pilot, year 2)

> *... there's no rocket science in PMS, it's just GMS under a different name.*
>
> (practice-based pilot, year 3)

Does it matter that, in clinical terms at least, PMS appears to differ so little from GMS? While PMS pilots were set the task of improving fairness, efficiency, effectiveness, responsiveness, integration, flexibility and accountability, it was not the intention that they would, necessarily, provide a wholly different clinical service. This view was summed up by one of the GPs we interviewed who, in comparing her registered population with that of neighbouring practices, commented:

> *I think there are differences, and it's in terms of who we've got registered as opposed, necessarily, to what we do with them.*

Conclusions

More than 100 PMS pilots were approved to 'go live' in April 1998, with extremely high expectations that they would be able to deliver changes to traditional ways of working in primary care, and all this within a three-year timescale. As the four pilots taking part in the King's Fund evaluation have made clear, the early years of the pilots' lives were spent putting systems in place and building relationships with other organisations. Despite achieving high scores for a number of quality indicators (most notably the angina audit and practice profile questionnaire), there is no compelling evidence that PMS delivers higher quality simply because it is PMS. Ultimately, three years has proved too short a timeframe to judge the ability of the pilots to achieve their own objectives. This may seem slow progress; however, this period has been one of huge organisational change that has impacted not only on the pilots themselves, but also on all local stakeholders. Effort that would otherwise have been devoted to the pilot has been diverted to other tasks.

The pilots and the individuals involved have taken risks in setting up new and innovative services, in all cases drawing flak from a number of quarters. The trail-blazing nature of pilots and their enthusiasm have had an impact on the growth of later PMS initiatives. While the pilots were seen as being courageous in their willingness to 'stick their necks out', many of our respondents felt that the services they were providing were not so very different from more traditional GMS services. The trust-led pilots did, however, feel that they had been successful in attracting those marginalised groups of patients they had set out to recruit, thus increasing accessibility.

Patients appeared to rate the trust-led sites more critically than respondents at the practice-based sites, but there may be a number of explanations for this. One of the trust-led pilots was described as being '… about accessing groups of patients that have never been accessed before using a model of delivery that's never been used before'. Such pilots set out in extremely challenging circumstances to establish brand new practices in socially deprived areas. Anecdotal evidence suggests that patients registering with these practices have high levels of need and, in one of the pilots in particular, a large number of the patients are refugees and asylum seekers. GPAS, the questionnaire with which we measured levels of patient satisfaction with primary care services, was written in English and unlikely to be completed by non-English-speaking, highly mobile populations. Additional data collection to explore the satisfaction with services of these groups would be valuable.

The four pilots all felt that they had built solid foundations in setting up relationships with other organisations, an achievement that proved to be of benefit to the pilots themselves, and also to the collaborating organisations.

Timing of data collection is clearly a critical issue in any evaluation. 'Snapshots' of particular moments in practices' development may serve to highlight transitional difficulties that may subsequently be resolved, and may not be typical of future experiences. Despite the sometimes negative messages given by staff we interviewed in the PMS pilots themselves, by the final year of the evaluation the overall feeling emerging from the practice-based pilots was that, after 'treading water' in the early stages, pilots were now making progress and 'coming about very gradually'. The pace of change and resultant workloads in the trust-led pilots were often described as 'overwhelming'. However, these pilots were extremely positive about having reached their target populations.

Box 1.1 EDITH CAVELL PRACTICE, LAMBETH

Located in a community trust-owned building in Streatham Hill, an area of inner London with high levels of socio-economic deprivation, the Edith Cavell opened its doors for new patient registration in September 1998. The local community trust, Lambeth Healthcare NHS Trust (now Community Health South London NHS Trust) had identified a 'gap' in the provision of general practice services to a number of groups such as refugees, asylum seekers, the homeless and drug users. Primary care services in the area were fragmented, with many small practices, and provision was described as being of 'patchy quality and under significant pressure' (bid document), and there was anecdotal evidence that patients were experiencing difficulties in registering at local practices.

Based on their experience of providing nurse-led services to homeless people across the three boroughs of Lambeth, Southwark and Lewisham, the community trust was keen that the new practice should be set up as one of only ten nurse-led first wave PMS pilots in the country. The trust estimated that, once the pilot was underway, no more than 20 or 30 per cent of patients would need any direct input from the GP. The pilot was given the go-ahead to 'go live' by the Secretary of State for Health, and a lead nurse and two job-share GPs came into post in the summer and autumn of 1998 respectively.

Although patient registration did not happen as quickly as had been anticipated, by the end of the first year the practice had 1134 patients on its list. In April 2000, the community trust took on the list of a former single-handed practice co-located within the same building, and launched this as a second wave pilot, which increased the total Edith Cavell list to almost 5000 patients. While practice staff are confident that their practice is reaching the marginalised groups of patients they had intended to target, the practice has experienced some difficulties over the past three years, most notably in the negotiation of the respective roles of nurses, doctors and administrative staff. Staff turnover at the site has been very high and none of the original staff involved in the setting up of the pilot remain. At the time of writing, the distinctive nurse-led focus of the pilot is being reconsidered.

Box 1.2 Isleworth Centre Practice

Like the Edith Cavell Practice, the Isleworth Centre Practice was set up as a greenfield practice by a community trust in a relatively deprived area of London. Hounslow and Spelthorne Community Mental Health Trust had identified an area of Isleworth in which primary care provision had failed to keep pace with the rapid population growth and, according to anecdotal evidence, patients were experiencing difficulty in registering with local practices. At the time the PMS pilot bid document was written, there were no other GP practices in the two wards of Isleworth North and Isleworth South, with a combined population of 20,000 people, and the nearest health centre was three miles away.

The trust planned that the PMS pilot, located in the premises of a former local authority day care centre for older people that had closed due to lack of funding, would provide a wider range of services than a more traditional GMS practice. After being given permission to go live in April 1998, the practice, which employed two job-share GPs, a nurse practitioner and a range of other staff, opened its doors in September 1998.

Patient registration was rapid, with up to 80 patients a week being registered at the outset, suggesting that the practice had targeted a genuine local need. By the end of the first 12 months, the total list size stood at 1300 patients. Patient demand was so great that the practice unwillingly decided to close its list temporarily to allow the team to 'draw breath' and, when the list was re-opened a few weeks later, a stricter set of registration criteria was instituted. In January 2001, the list size stood at 1994 patients. Like the Edith Cavell Practice, turnover of staff was high, with both job-share GPs leaving the practice after the first year.

The community trust consulted widely at the bid stage of the project, involving a large number of community and voluntary groups, and thus gave 'people power' to the project, which was also based on a public health needs assessment carried out in the area. A number of other organisations were co-located within the building.

Box 1.3 SOUTH WEST LONDON PRIMARY CARE ORGANISATION

Eight south London practices with a history of working together as fundholding practices, and subsequently as a total purchasing pilot (TPP), submitted a successful bid in 1997 to become a first wave PMS pilot. With 44 GPs working from 12 surgery premises, serving a population of 81,000 patients across the three boroughs of Merton, Sutton and Wandsworth, the practices, though not entirely geographically contiguous, nevertheless shared the same broad aims and objectives.

One of the practices left the PMS pilot at the end of the first 12 months as its catchment area was not coterminous with the eventual, and much debated, PCG configuration in the area. The remaining seven practices formalised their *de facto* partnership, and changed the Companies Act in the process, by becoming the largest single GP partnership in the country. In April 2000, the PCG within which the PMS was situated became one of the first PCTs in the country, and in July 1999 the remaining 12 non-PMS practices within the PCT area heard that they had been successful in their bid to become a second wave PMS pilot – making the Nelson and West Merton PCT a whole-PMS PCT.

Although the PMS pilot serves a largely affluent area, a number of areas were identified in which staff wished to institute quality improvements to the services they provided. They hoped to build on the intermediate care project (an initiative of the TPP) in order to provide secondary care services in the community, particularly to older people. The appointment of a mental health adviser and the setting up of the mental health project were similarly planned to extend the provision of services to the severely mentally ill in the community. Other innovations planned included a reduction in the level of administration in general practice, and the development of integrated pathways for the management of chronic conditions.

Summing up the developments over the first three years of the pilot's life, staff felt that much time had been lost in the negotiations around PCG configuration and in the move to PCT status. While describing the early years of the pilot as simply 'treading water', there was a feeling that, by the end of year three, the pilot was 'coming back to life'.

Box 1.4 North Hillingdon PMS Pilot

Made up of three practices – one group and two single-handed – the North Hillingdon PMS Pilot is situated in Ruislip, an affluent area of north-west London. In applying to become a first wave PMS pilot, the practices planned to work more closely together, using a new, more collaborative, organisational model to provide more coherence to the services they had previously provided independently. The key aims of the pilot were to:

- increase capacity by attracting appropriate general practitioner and nursing resources
- share clinical and management resources
- make better use of skill mix and develop a team approach to service delivery
- improve the management of specific patient groups such as older patients
- reduce individual practice administrative workload.

The group practice had computerised all practice notes, and felt that this would increase accessibility for patients who could now be seen at either the main or the branch surgery. Staff in this pilot were extremely enthusiastic about the potential of working more closely together. Though this had been achieved to some extent, they acknowledged that there was more work to be done in building inter-practice collaboration.

Relationships between the pilot and the health authority have not always been cordial, and the pilot contract was signed late because of difficulties in agreeing contract detail. However, both practice and health authority felt that relationships between the two had improved recently.

Difficulties in funding had been a feature of this pilot since the outset, and this delayed the launch of the elderly care project. However, there was a feeling that things were getting moving again in year three.

References

1 Department of Health. *Personal medical services pilots under the NHS (Primary Care) Act 1997: a guide to local evaluation.* London: NHSE, 1997.

2 Jenkins C, Lewis R, Gillam S. *Isleworth Centre Practice Personal Medical Services (PMS) Pilot: King's Fund evaluation report April 1998–March 2001.* London: King's Fund, 2001.

3 Jenkins C, Lewis R, Gillam S. *Edith Cavell Practice Personal Medical Services (PMS) Pilot: King's Fund evaluation report April 1998–March 2001.* London: King's Fund, 2001.

4 Jenkins C, Lewis R, Gillam S. *South West London Primary Care Organisation Personal Medical Services (PMS) Pilot: King's Fund evaluation report April 1998–March 2001.* London: King's Fund, 2001.

5 Jenkins C, Lewis R, Gillam S. *North Hillingdon Personal Medical Services (PMS) Pilot: King's Fund evaluation report April 1998–March 2001.* London: King's Fund, 2001.

6 Lewis R, Gillam S, Gosden R, Sheaff R. Who contracts for primary care? *Journal of Public Health Medicine* 1999; 21: 367–71.

7 Airey C, Bruster S, Erens B, Lilley S-J, Pickering K, Pitson L. *National surveys of NHS patients: general practice 1998.* London: NHSE, 1999.

8 Campbell S, Roland M, Buetow S. Defining quality of care. *Social Science and Medicine* 2000; 51: 1611–25.

9 Ramsay J, Campbell J L, Schroter S, Green J, Roland M. The general practice assessment survey (GPAS): tests of data quality and measurement properties. *Family Practice* 2000; 17: 372–9.

10 Quality of Care Project (TQP) for the National Evaluation of Primary Care Act Personal Medical Services Pilots. *Does PMS improve the quality of care? Interim report to the Department of Health.* Southampton: University of Southampton, 2000.

11 Hunjan M, Edwards J. *Isleworth Centre Practice: local evaluation of consultation pattern and financial status – interim report.* London: Ealing, Hammersmith and Hounslow Health Authority/Isleworth Centre Practice, 2001.

12 NPCRDC. *National evaluation of first wave personal medical services pilots: integrated interim report from four research projects.* Manchester: NPCRDC, 2000.

13 Department of Health. *Personal medical services pilots under the NHS (Primary Care) Act 1997: a comprehensive guide.* London: NHSE, 1997.

14 Department of Health. *Personal medical services pilots under the NHS (Primary Care) Act 1997: a comprehensive guide.* 2nd edition. London: NHSE, 1998.

15 Walsh N, André C, Barnes M, Huntingdon J, Rogers H, Baines D. *New opportunities for primary care? A second year report of first wave PMS pilots in England.* Birmingham: Health Services Management Centre, 2000.

16 National Primary Care Research and Development Centre (Chapple A, MacDonald W, Rogers A, Sergison M.). *Can nurses replace GPs? An evaluation of a nurse-led personal medical services pilot scheme.* Manchester: NPCRDC, 1999.

17 Lewis R. *Nurse-led primary care: learning from PMS pilots.* London: King's Fund, 2001.

18 Hunjan M, Edwards J. *Isleworth Centre Practice: local evaluation of consultation pattern and financial status – interim report.* London: Ealing, Hammersmith and Hounslow Health Authority/Isleworth Centre Practice, 2001.

Chapter 2

Nurse-led PMS pilots

Richard Lewis

Introduction

In announcing a first wave of PMS pilots, Frank Dobson, then Secretary of State for Health, specifically encouraged nurses to use them as an opportunity to develop a new kind of primary care: a primary care that maximised the nursing contribution as well as the leadership qualities of nurses themselves. Subsequently, nine 'nurse-led' pilots were approved to begin operation on 1 April 1998. This chapter summarises the findings of a King's Fund evaluation of these pilots and considers the experience of 'nurse leadership' so far.[1]

Tony Blair challenged the health service to 'strip out unnecessary demarcations, introduce more flexible training and working practices, and ensure that doctors do not use time dealing with patients who could be treated safely by other health care staff'.[2] Health Secretary Alan Milburn, in his address to the Annual Congress of the Royal College of Nursing in 2000, stressed that nurses were at the centre of the Government's plans for modernisation, and promised 'a health service which liberates nurses not limits them'.[3]

The Secretary of State identified ten nurse roles that should, in future, become widespread throughout the NHS – later described as the Chief Nursing Officer's 'ten key roles for nurses' (see Box 2.1). These roles built on the experience and achievements of leaders in the field; if opportunities to fulfil these roles were available to some then they should be available to all – appropriately skilled – nurses. Nurses of the future look set to move into territory hitherto firmly occupied by doctors.

This theme of shuffling the professional pack was one that was embellished in the NHS Plan. The post-Plan NHS was to be responsive, convenient and tailored to individual needs. Access to primary and

---

Box 2.1 THE CHIEF NURSING OFFICER'S TEN KEY ROLES FOR NURSES

- order diagnostic investigations (e.g. pathology tests and X-rays)
- make and receive referrals direct (e.g. to a therapist or pain consultant)
- admit and discharge patients for specified conditions and within agreed protocols
- manage patient caseloads (e.g. for diabetes and rheumatology)
- run clinics (e.g. ophthalmology and dermatology)
- prescribe medicines and treatment
- carry out a wide range of resuscitation procedures, including defibrillation
- perform minor surgery and outpatient procedures
- triage patients using the latest IT to the most appropriate health professional
- take a lead in the way local health services are organised and in the way they are run.

---

intermediate care services was particularly highlighted. Nurses were to act as linchpins of this new NHS. According to the Government, 'pressure on GP services will be eased as nurses and other community staff ... take on more tasks'.[4] Instant access to primary care advice via NHS Direct, rapid access within the GP surgery, the encouragement of GPs to develop sub-specialisms – all rely on nurses carrying out extended roles.

The nine nurse-led PMS pilots provide early learning in the development of extended nursing roles.

Evaluation methods

This evaluation focuses on the views and perceptions of the pilot nurse leads themselves. Therefore, the nine nurses (and in some cases their immediate managers, where they have been heavily involved in establishing the pilots) have provided the data upon which this report is based.

The main form of data collection has been through two focus groups (held in June and December 2000). Seven of the nine sites attended the first focus group and four sites were represented at the second. In addition, other data were collected by questionnaires completed by all sites and, where relevant, through reference to the wider King's Fund evaluation of PMS pilots (see previous chapter).

Pilot characteristics

Eight of the nine pilots were newly established practices, providing services where previously none had been provided (see Table 2.1 below). In one case, the nurse-led pilot was awarded a vacant list following the death of the incumbent GP. Six of the nine pilots were designed to provide services to specifically targeted populations (though not necessarily exclusively to these populations) or to increase access to primary care for the general population in 'under-doctored' areas. The most common population groups targeted were those of homeless people (five pilots) and refugees and asylum seekers (two pilots).

The nine pilots adopted one of three organisational and contractual approaches. The most common arrangement was for the pilot to be managed by a community NHS trust that held a contract with the local health authority (five pilots). Two pilots were managed by existing general practices that established branch surgeries or quasi-independent organisations. In one case, the contract holder was a PMS practice; in the other, a GMS practice. Finally, two pilots were provided by independently contracted nurses who contracted on their own behalf with their local health authority and directly employed practice staff.

Four of the nine pilots contracted to provide PMS Plus services (i.e. services that are beyond those provided as standard within a general practice). In three of these pilots, the 'Plus' element comprised community nursing services; in the fourth, child development and midwifery services.

Pilots were established with a wide range of individual objectives; however, a number of themes emerged across pilots. These included:

- serving vulnerable populations (5 pilots)
- providing 'patient-focused' or 'user-friendly' services (4 pilots)
- developing the clinical skills of team members and/or breaking down professional boundaries (4 pilots)

- improving patient access to primary care (4 pilots)
- community development and/or patient empowerment (4 pilots)
- developing partnerships with other agencies, and voluntary or community groups (2 pilots).

By December 2000 (two years and eight months after their intended start dates), the nine pilots displayed a wide range in the number of registered patients. List sizes ranged from 500 to 2600 patients, with a mean of 1311 patients. Some of the pilots with particularly low list sizes were serving well-defined populations with particularly high needs (for example, pilots serving exclusively homeless populations). In other cases, pilots had experienced a rapid on-take of patients since their establishment and were serving populations of 2000 or more.

The composition of the clinical teams also varies widely among pilots. There is no clear pattern between list size and size of the clinical team. In some cases, the ratio of clinicians to patients might be considered quite high compared to 'traditional' general practice. An 'average' GP principal is likely to have a registered list of 1845 patients. Each principal will, on average, work with 0.4 of a 'whole time equivalent' practice nurse.[5] Nurse-led PMS pilots tend to have a significantly 'richer' primary health care team, in terms of both the doctor–nurse ratio and the total clinical resource. However, it should be noted that the population served by the nine nurse-led pilots may be significantly different to the average and many are associated with significant deprivation and high health needs.

Defining 'nurse-led primary care'

The nurse leads have developed a multi-factorial understanding of what 'nurse-led primary care' means in practice. Interestingly, only part of this definition relates to the clinical contribution of the nurse lead. Nurse 'leadership' is as much a philosophical as it is a clinical construct.

Two distinct components of 'nurse-led primary care' can be identified within the context of PMS pilots:

- implementation of enhanced nursing roles
- a 'nurse-led' value system.

Implementation of enhanced nursing roles

Nurse leads emphasised that their pilots provided an opportunity to carry out extended nursing roles. The most important extended role is that of the clinical assessment and treatment of patients undifferentiated by need. The nurse leads described themselves as 'gatekeepers' and 'navigators' (terms usually ascribed within the NHS to the role of the GP). Therefore, this traditional GP role is being undertaken by (or at least shared with) nurses within the nine pilot sites.

> *Patients go to the GP because they don't know where else to go, and I put myself in the place of the first port of call so that I can maybe navigate or help that person. If it's me, that's fine; if it's the GP, that's fine. But it may be [the] marriage guidance [service].*

The nursing role of initial patient assessment (or 'triage') was also a hallmark of nurse-led care. However, this was carried out differently across the nine pilots. In some pilots, all urgent, same-day patient appointments are taken by the nurse lead; in others, patients may choose whether to see a nurse or a GP.

A 'nurse-led' value system

Nurse leads all emphasised that their pilots were based on an overt value system that renegotiated two sets of relationships: those between clinicians within the primary health care team and those between the team and its patients.

The relations between team members (particularly between nurses and doctors) are intended to reflect new values of equality and respect for complementary professional competencies. In part, this is intended to free nurses to use their skills to the full and to redress a power imbalance between doctors and nurses, allowing the latter to enjoy the autonomy so long enjoyed by the former:

> *It is about challenging how we have traditionally delivered the care and that has always been medically led ... it's about the acknowledgement that nurses can do that.*

Table 2.1 Characteristics of the first wave nurse-led PMS pilots

Pilot	Main characteristics	Service provider/ contract holder	Pilot aims	List size (1/12/00)	Staffing
Acorns	Services to travellers, the homeless and refugees in Thurrock. Offers outreach services. Many non-English-speaking patients.	South Essex Mental Health and Community NHS Trust	Target vulnerable patient groups. Redesign services to be more patient focused. Maximise competencies of nurses and doctors.	1000	NP – 1 WTE GP – 0.8 WTE
Appleton Primary Care	New practice in affluent part of Warrington. Focus on use of IT and patient partnership.	Warrington Community NHS Trust	Offer holistic and patient-focused services. Break down professional barriers. Offer 'good value'.	1000	NP – 1 WTE GP – 1 WTE PN – 1 WTE
Arch Day Centre	Branch surgery of existing GMS practice offering services to homeless people in Stoke.	PMS GP	Develop services for vulnerable young people. Increase access and provide user-friendly environment. Client participation. Partnership and collaboration with statutory and voluntary sector groups.	350 + 50 temp resident	NP – 1 WTE GP (as required) Substance misuse clinician *GP input provided by linked PMS practice*
Daruzzaman Care Centre	Replacement of existing GMS practice in Salford on death of GP.	Independent nurse contractor	Offer patient-focused care. Emphasis on community/social priorities. Value access, flexibility, choice and empowerment.	1950	NP – 1 WTE GP – 2 WTE covering clinical, audit, training and research duties

Practice	Description	Provider	Aims	List size	Staffing
Edith Cavell Practice*	New practice offering services to vulnerable groups (refugees, homeless, mentally ill, substance abusers). Now also providing wave 2 pilot.	Community Health South London NHS Trust	Improving access and services for vulnerable groups. Higher quality via structured approach to care. Close working with community groups. Develop links with RCN institute.	2600 (W1 pilot)*	NP (1 WTE) GP (1.5 WTE)
Meadowfields Practice	New practice in Derby.	Independent nurse contractor	Shift in power-base from GPs to wider team. Patients to be seen by most appropriate clinician. Involvement of patients in service design.	2500	PN (lead) – 1 WTE GP – 1.25 WTE PN – 0.8 WTE
Morley Street Surgery	New practice in Brighton providing services to homeless people, including outreach services. Working in partnership with a range of voluntary and statutory agencies.	South Downs Health Trust	Target vulnerable patients. Enhanced NP role. Team-based approach with wider range of expertise within the team.	847	NP – 1 WTE GP – 1.3 WTE
The Spitalfields PMS Practice	PMS branch of a GMS practice providing services to homeless people in E1 and the City.	The Spitalfields Practice (GMS)	Target homeless populations – street homeless – hostel homeless	500	NP – 2 WTE GP – 1 WTE
Valley Park Surgery	New surgery offering services to under-doctored area.	Croydon and Surrey Downs Community NHS Trust	Improved access. Emphasis on community development.	1000	NP/HV – 0.8 WTE PN – 1 WTE GP – 0.4 WTE GP input contracted from PCG

* These figures relate to a first wave pilot. The Edith Cavell Practice has also undertaken a second wave pilot.

GP = general practitioner   NP = nurse practitioner   PN = practice nurse

This desire to challenge the perceived *status quo* emerged from strongly held perceptions among the nurse leads that the professional culture of nurses was less conservative and more willing to promote patients' interests than that of traditional general practice. Nurse leads also emphasised the importance of the non-profit-making nature of their pilots. This they contrasted with the incentives that existed for GPs under the GMS contract.

Their philosophy was underpinned by a belief that they had established a significantly different relationship with their patients. This reflected a mission to empower patients and to locate the work of the practices within the wider community, taking account of patients' social concerns. Nurse leads emphasised their willingness to offer patients choice and responsibility in relation to their care. While nurse leads accepted that a minority of GMS practices aspired to a similar vision, they nevertheless associated patient empowerment and inter-professional equality with nursing, rather than medical values and culture. Doctors that concurred with this view were described by one lead as 'closet nurses'.

In many respects, therefore, the defining characteristic of the nurse-led pilots is not concerned with 'leadership' by nurses at all, but by an equality of opportunity, mutual respect among team members and a focus on the needs of patients. In these respects, the title 'nurse-led' may be misleading, although it clearly has important symbolic value.

PMS – reaching the parts not reached by GMS

Perhaps not surprisingly, given their philosophy, the nurse-led pilots are strongly associated with vulnerable, or traditionally under-served, populations. Seven of the nine pilots were established in response to the needs of particular types of patients (such as the homeless and refugees) or to serve areas with generally inadequate access to primary care services.

This association between PMS pilots and deprivation or particular patient needs has been remarked upon before[6,7] and features among the governmental aims set out for PMS.[8] Therefore, this aspect of the nurse-led pilots may stem from their inclusion within the PMS movement in general, rather than from their nurse-led orientation. However, it is notable that a far greater proportion of nurse-led pilots are seeking to fill the gaps left by GMS than is true for PMS pilots as a whole. Are nurse-led services particularly suited to this type of work? Nurse leads feel that they are. In particular, they suggest that nursing culture and skills appear well suited to working within complex social and clinical environments, and in promoting wider public health within communities (although many primary care doctors might well claim the same thing).

Nurse leads contrast starkly their new model of care with that of 'traditional' general practice:

> We did manage to work in a different way … which was very different to anything … I've done before; going out into the community and finding [out what] people needed and … getting feedback from them rather than just providing a service that we thought was appropriate.

One consequence of the emergence of these new types of pilot appears to be a growing division between services for vulnerable populations and mainstream primary care. Nurse-led pilots have a tendency to act as beacons for particular patient groups, drawing them away from other practices. Nurse leads were aware that neighbouring practices may also deliberately direct certain of their own registered patients (or people seeking to register) towards the new service:

> Our local GPs now would say [to patients] … 'Go to that practice', and that's fine because in many respects they would get a better deal from us anyway because we are tailored and hopefully more responsive to their need than the other practice populations in the locality.

While the advantage to patients who register with practices that are willing and able to care for them is self-evident, it raises an uncomfortable issue of restricted patient choice. If other general practices in the area feel able to divest themselves of responsibilities towards certain population groups, these patients may effectively have a choice of only one source of primary care. Similarly, the spectre of general practices 'picking and choosing' patients sits uneasily with the vision of a comprehensive health service offering equal access to all. This potential for 'ghetto primary care', also raised by Clare Jenkins in the previous chapter, is not restricted to the 'nurse-led' model of care.

Pushing back the professional boundaries?

Significantly, nurse leads expressed serious reservations about the way in which extended nursing roles in primary care had been introduced and the feasibility of their wider promulgation within the NHS. Of particular concern was the rise in the popularity of the nurse practitioner role (or, at least, the use of that title) and the relative lack of regulation and quality control over the practice of these nurses. Nurse leads drew attention to the fact that no nationally agreed competencies, standards or training curricula exist for the role of 'nurse practitioner', and were critical of the United Kingdom Central Council (the, now reformed, nursing regulatory body) for this omission.

> *People have done a three-day course or a six-day course or a six-week course and call themselves [a nurse practitioner]. There is no underpinning for it, there is no basic standard and we need to have that laid down, so that nationally there is the same standard applied.*

While clinical governance processes at local level are intended to provide a quality assurance framework for the work of the nurse-led pilots, the experience of the nurse leads suggests that this is, so far, ineffective:

> *You end up with a clinical governance lead who says … 'Well, we won't bother coming to you because you are so far above the rest we have to concentrate on those who aren't' … So nobody is doing any clinical governance with us; we haven't had a visit.*

Nurse leads recognised that their position as 'pioneers' of new nursing roles made them a potent symbol for nurses elsewhere. However, they were concerned that the next cadre of nurse leads was not materialising – they know of only a trickle of nurses that might join them. In part, they ascribed this reticence among nurses to step into nurse-led roles as a response to the difficulties the nine pilots had faced in establishing their pilots.

Inter-professional relations

The nurse leads' vision of inter-professional equality and co-operation has been discussed. To what extent has this vision found its expression in reality?

In many pilots, the internal team dynamics were consistent with the vision. However, in a minority of pilots some conflicts of power emerged between doctors and nurses within the pilots. At its most benign this manifested itself through GP control of the management of patient care, in particular retaining the power of deciding which clinician would see which patient. The existing legal framework (particularly that patients can be registered only with a doctor, that a doctor must be present whenever patients are treated, and the current requirement that GPs must sign virtually all prescriptions) has undermined the nurses' ability to manage the pilots independently.

Where relationships between medical and nursing team members were good, and where they shared a common vision of practice, this problem has been overcome. In most pilots, doctors and nurse leads worked hard together to implement flexible systems. However, in one pilot significant problems emerged within the team over the interpretation of 'nurse-led' services and over the respective roles of doctors and nurses within the pilot:

> So in terms of professions working more closely together, actually we were doctors and nurses at war in the end; worse than in any other job I'd been in.

This pilot saw the rapid departure of two nurse leads within two years of its inception.

While good inter-professional relations could generally be maintained within pilots, nurse leads experienced a significant degree of suspicion and sometimes hostility from neighbouring GPs and Local Medical Committees (LMCs). One focus of this hostility was the employment of salaried GPs. Nurse leads perceived the concerns of local doctors (particularly LMCs) to stem mainly from concerns that salaried general practice would undermine the system of GMS and represented the 'thin end of the wedge'. This has been reported elsewhere[9] and appears to be an issue related to PMS pilots generally, rather than to nurse-led pilots specifically.

However, some scepticism by local doctors about the actual model of nurse-led care was also reported. This may well have heightened the local hostility felt towards the pilots. This is explored further by Catherine Baraniak and Lance Gardner in Chapter 5).

Nurse leads also questioned whether inter-professional tension was heightened if nurse-led pilots sought to provide mainstream services, rather than a service aimed at vulnerable groups poorly served by GMS:

> When we tried to get a PMS pilot for the ordinary population, we were stopped by the medics ... all of a sudden we were encroaching on what was traditionally their territory ... to say I got assassinated by the medical colleagues ... was an understatement.

Notwithstanding these early difficulties, nurse leads also reported that the sense of hostility and isolation that they felt diminished as the number of PMS pilots increased nationally. Again, this is consistent with other evaluation findings that suggest that, over time, tensions between pilots and primary care colleagues have dissipated.[10]

The primary–secondary care interface

A key attribute for nurse-led primary care is that nurses can directly access diagnostic services and make and receive referrals from the hospital sector. This is also set out as one of the Chief Nursing Officer's ten challenges for nurses (see Box 2.1).

The experience of nurse leads in implementing this has been varied. While some hospitals have responded quickly to the changes imposed upon them by primary care, others have proved more inflexible. Only two pilots have negotiated formal arrangements with hospital NHS trusts. The majority relies on informal arrangements agreed with individual hospital clinicians and departments. These arrangements have evolved and, over time, led to a gradual extension of the range of specialties prepared to accept referrals from nurse leads. However, few nurse leads can expect a standard response from their hospital providers and may have to undertake substantial work to develop relationships that support the philosophy of their pilot. This has been successful in many cases and some consultants have undertaken a significant culture change.

> *Any referral I send comes back to me personally and I have a relationship with the consultants which two years ago, they say, there is no way [they] would have got into.*

Where problems existed, they were likely to reflect distrust by particular hospital staff, and the response of hospital departments and individual consultants was markedly different.

> *Every X-ray now gets phoned up to see if the doctors saw it or the nurse … some of the labs are OK, but not ultrasound. The same applies to microbiology. It has caused a huge problem because all they keep doing is sending stuff back saying, 'Doctor unknown.'*

Yet, despite their problems, nurse leads do not necessarily interpret consultant behaviour as simple professional intransigence. They have considerable sympathy with what they see as a professional dilemma for consultants. This stems from their concerns about the lack of recognised standards and competencies that underpin the role of nurse practitioner. Consultants, they argue, are not able to judge the validity of any referral that they receive from a nurse practitioner.

Implementing the pilots – 'swimming against the tide'

All nurse leads emphasised the struggles that they had undergone in implementing their pilots. Introducing a radical new model of service has not been achieved easily. Many of the obstacles they faced were bureaucratic. The automatic response of the NHS was to expect that the roles undertaken by the nurse leads would, instead, be carried out by doctors. Nurse leads were trying to change '50 years of history' and felt they were 'wading through treacle'.

A number of issues relating to implementation emerged.

Regulatory obstacles

Nurse leads identified a range of regulatory obstacles that hindered them from fulfilling their roles. The signatures of primary care nurses are not acceptable to the Benefits Agency in relation to absence from work due to sickness, nor are they accepted on death certificates. As Catherine Baraniak and Lance Gardner describe later, this can cause inconvenience and upset for patients.

Of perhaps greater significance is the highly restricted ability of nurses to prescribe pharmaceuticals. While the ability to prescribe is critical to their work, nurse leads all felt that their current scope (under the existing nurse prescribing scheme) was minimal and inadequate. Nurse-led pilots have developed informal arrangements with the GPs in their teams, whereby prescriptions are routinely signed having been drawn up by the nurse lead. This may or may not include a clinical review of the patient's notes by the GP prior to signing. Nurse leads have been careful to prepare prescriptions only within their own competencies. Even so, any GP signing such a prescription is felt to be, in the words of one nurse lead, 'on the boundaries of legality'.

Project sponsors and local champions

Five of the nine pilots are sponsored and managed by community NHS trusts. Many of these trusts established the schemes out of a desire to push back professional boundaries and to offer services to previously under-served populations. Notwithstanding their motivations, nurse leads identified some disadvantages associated with community trust-managed schemes.

In particular, nurse leads identified a lack of autonomy over the management of their pilot and felt themselves the victims of an excessive bureaucracy. Community trusts were perceived as generally ignorant about the operational detail of general practice, nor could they respond rapidly to the day-to-day needs of primary care organisations. As public bodies, they had a considerable bureaucracy that could not be sidestepped:

> *Our fridge broke down and I was four weeks without a fridge because*
> *Electrolux wouldn't send me a new fridge because the trust had not paid*
> *for it … Had I been in my previous practice and managed by a GP …*
> *he would've said, 'There's a cheque, go get a fridge.'*

However, it cannot be inferred from this that the independent contractor
or general practice model of a pilot necessarily provides a more
satisfactory vehicle. Independent contractor nurse leads commented that
their position, while maximising autonomy, provided few, if any,
mechanisms for their own personal support. The independent contractor
model of nurse-led primary care can result in isolation, often in the face
of considerable resistance or hostility to the work that he or she is trying
to undertake.

Nurse leads identified that local champions were important to the success
of any pilot. Within a trust-managed pilot, operational managers have
been able to support and encourage nurse leads. This has been seen as a
means to minimise stress on the nurse lead (although it has not been
perceived as forthcoming in all the trust-managed pilots).

It appears, therefore, that nurse leads face a trade-off between autonomy
and personal support. Trust-managed pilots may provide greater personal
support to their nurse leads, but at the cost of an inadequate management
support service. Independent contractor nurses are able to manage their
own organisations, but must face any resistance to their pilot largely
alone (though health authorities have, in some cases, provided support).
The issue of support is significant: nurse leads clearly feel that they face a
degree of exposure far greater than that experienced by other health
professionals.

Conclusion

More than three years into their pilots, the nine nurse-led pilots have
achieved a great deal. New practices have been formed, many thousands
of patients are being served, and nurses have been responsible for
developing and leading teams of primary care professionals. In a very real
sense, the nurse-led PMS pilots are putting in place the radical vision for
health care called for by Tony Blair and his government.

And yet these developments have not been without personal costs for the nurses involved. A punishing workload and a highly politicised environment, with resistance or blockages from many quarters, appear to have been the norm. Certainly the NHS juggernaut will not turn on a sixpence. Nor should the 'forces of conservatism' be underestimated: nurse leads have faced professional and bureaucratic obstacles that have proved quite unyielding.

What can we learn from their experiences? First, nurse-led primary care is about more than changing professional roles. The nurse leads have aspired to create a service and a culture that has patient needs and inter-professional equality at its centre. This transcends any model of 'nurse leadership' and even PMS itself. This philosophy has always had its adherents within GMS; perhaps PMS makes it more easy to achieve.

Second, the model of enhanced nursing roles is not without controversy; certainly, the medical jury is still out, and local doctors in particular were suspicious. Nurse leadership is but one further change heralded by PMS pilots that have, more generally, raised the hackles of a section of 'traditional' general practice.

Yet it would be wrong to overplay the resistance faced by the pilots – pilots made good progress in winning referral rights within their local hospitals. However, this was not universal and remains mainly an informal arrangement, with some consultants feeling able to ignore the reality of the extended nursing role. These consultants still prefer to communicate only with other doctors.

Third, the provision of dedicated services for vulnerable population groups raises some interesting ethical issues. PMS pilots have proved popular because they are sympathetic and skilled in dealing with particular patient groups. However, as a consequence GMS practices are perceived to direct refugees or homeless people to PMS practices rather than accept them onto their own lists. Is this simply a sensible use of scarce skills or is it the creation of 'ghetto primary care'?

Fourth, the issue of excessive bureaucracy was raised. In part, this relates to NHS and welfare regulations that do not recognise the new role of nurses in primary care. These regulations should be amended (in the case of nurse prescribing, a liberalisation of the current legal framework is imminent). More worrying, perhaps, was the bureaucracy associated with NHS trust management of PMS pilots. As these trusts are transformed into PCTs, what does this tell us about the future for PCT-led PMS pilots?

PCTs, with primary care at their heart, might be expected to have a greater degree of knowledge of (and perhaps sympathy for) the day-to-day needs of PMS practices, whether nurse-led or not. Whether they will be able to overcome the tendency to bureaucratic inertia, so common in large organisations, is another matter – PCTs may not be any quicker to purchase the new practice refrigerator. Will PCTs be sympathetic to the aims of nurse-led pilots? Again, it is too early to say. PCTs may certainly share the vision of needs-led services, but will they want to challenge the power balance between GPs and nurses?

Lastly, and perhaps most importantly, do we have the right infrastructure to take forward a new model of primary care nursing? Nurse leads had significant concerns about the free use of the term 'nurse practitioner' and cast doubt on the training and competencies that currently underpin that role. As leading nurse practitioners themselves, this message should give pause for thought. Nurse leads raised the spectre of inadequate quality control and monitoring, both locally at practice level and nationally by professional bodies. Certainly, they appeared to receive little external professional support as they developed new and personally demanding roles.

So what can we deduce about the Government's strategy to increase the contribution of nurses as part of a new approach to 'demand management'? There is now a welter of evidence which supports the view that nurses are able successfully to carry out extended clinical roles at acceptable cost and with high patient satisfaction. The gradually emerging evidence base in relation to PMS pilots suggests that they provide a good vehicle for allowing nurses to innovate and to carry out new roles.[11,12] Other evaluations of nurse-led PMS pilots suggest that patients and practice staff are willing and able to embrace this new model with enthusiasm (though evidence about the cost-effectiveness of this model is, so far, unavailable).[13,14]

If we can tentatively conclude that nurse-led pilots have begun to deliver a new model of care, however, a further question is raised – are the nurses necessary for the Government's 'new NHS' available? Nurse leads doubted that they were. Clearly, both the medical and nursing professions are facing a crisis in recruitment. However, the perceived lack of successors to the first wave of nurse leads may also be a reflection of the difficulties experienced by the pioneers. As one lead commented:

> I'm not sure I would advise anyone to do it really, sadly. At this stage I think there are a lot more things that would need to change before it can be successful.

Nurse leads may prove to be a vanguard without an army.

References

1   Lewis R. *Nurse-led primary care: learning from PMS pilots*. London: King's Fund, 2001.
2   Blair T. Speech to House of Commons, 22 March 2000.
3   Milburn A. Speech to the Annual Congress of the Royal College of Nurses, 5 April 2000.
4   Secretary of State for Health. *The NHS Plan: a plan for investment; a plan for reform*. Cm 4818-I. London: The Stationery Office, 1997.
5   Department of Health. *Statistical Bulletin – Statistics for general medical practitioners in England: 1989–1999*. London: Department of Health, 2000.
6   Jenkins C, Lewis R. Reducing inequality. In: Lewis R, Gillam S, editors. *Transforming primary care: personal medical services in the new NHS*. London: King's Fund, 1999.
7   Carter Y, Curtis S, Harding G, Maguire A, Meads G, Riley A, Ross P, Underwood M. Addressing inequalities. In: *National evaluation of first wave NHS personal medical services pilots: integrated interim report from four research projects*. Manchester: NPCRDC, 2000.
8   Department of Health. *Personal medical services: application process for third wave pilots*. (HSC 2000/018). London: Department of Health, 2000.
9   Lewis R, Jenkins C, Gillam S. *Personal medical services pilots in London – rewriting the Red Book*. London: King's Fund, 1999.
10 Walsh N, Allen L, Baines D, Barnes M. *Taking off: a first year report of the personal medical services (PMS) pilots in England*. Birmingham: HSMC, 1999.
11 Walsh N, Huntington J. Testing the pilots. *Nursing Times* 2000; 96 (33): 32–3.

12 Walsh N, André C, Barnes M, Huntington J, Rogers H, Baines D. *New opportunities for primary care? A second year report of first wave PMS pilots in England.* Birmingham: HSMC, 2000.

13 Chapple A, Rogers A, Macdonald W, Sergison M. Patients' perceptions of changing professional boundaries and the future of 'nurse-led' services. *Primary Health Care Research and Development* 2000; 1: 51–9.

14 Chapple A, Sergison M. Challenging tradition. *Nursing Times* 1999; 95 (12): 32–3.

Section two

Chapter 3

Employing salaried GPs – Wolverhampton's experience

Tim Crossley

KEY POINTS

The Wolverhampton PMS project involves nine practices employed by the community trust. This flexible model of externally managed, salaried practice has helped to address recruitment and retention problems in a particularly deprived part of the city.

Why do doctors dislike salaries?

Doctors have always relished their freedom and GPs have maintained autonomy by not having a direct employer. In the profession's view, this has ensured an effective service in most of the country and flexible working conditions. GPs feel their role as patient advocate is more effective if they are independent of the State as well. They fear that salaried employment would mean more constraining terms and conditions.

But there are deeper psychological reasons why doctors cherish the sense that they can do as they see fit for their patients. Decision-making is lonely, and risk management in primary care creates anxiety. Doctors cope by working within the limitations of their knowledge base and personal thresholds for risk – familiar internal territory that they have evolved. Doctors do not wish to be told by managers, for instance, that drug A must now be used in preference to drug B, which he or she has grown to understand and like – it adds yet more uncertainty. So, formularies are not easily imposed. Likewise with appointment lengths, numbers of staff, liaison with the hospital, and other decisions affecting patients over which GPs exercise discretion.

Doctors, like all other workers, want a sense of control and, to employ doctors successfully, this has to be acknowledged. The wider demands of public accountability, clinical governance and our legal and cultural framework conspire to constrain the freedom the anxious doctor craves.

Primary Care Act freedoms

The 1997 NHS (Primary Care) Act that introduced PMS pilots was more enabling of innovation than was understood by many GPs at the time. The Act granted the freedom to negotiate a better service locally by separating the roles of contractor and doctor. The first wave was further encouraged to redefine the GP's role.

However, the financial principle was established that a PMS practice should not cost more to run than a GMS practice providing the same service. The Act was seen by most of the profession's representative bodies as retrograde. First, changing from a national to a local contract meant the British Medical Association (BMA) and its General Practice Committee (GPC) lost 'influence'. A significant campaign to discourage GPs from changing their terms of service was launched. Behind much of this lay the fear of loss of independent contractor status. Interestingly, as it turned out the great majority of GPs working under PMS chose to remain with a profit-sharing system rather than opt for a salary.

Wolverhampton's problems and the scheme that emerged

Wolverhampton includes areas of extreme deprivation. Primary care provision in such an environment has always been difficult: recruitment is hard, and the levels of morbidity and workload are high. The deprivation payment scheme introduced in 1990 did not improve recruitment. Its 63 practices, 30 of them single handed, served a population of over 250,000. Governments and health authorities have tended to promote a belief in the efficiency and quality of group practice. Various attempts to manage small practices were made. Yet as fast as single-handed vacancies were given to partnerships, group practices split up, leaving the number of single-handed doctors stable. The population of GPs was ageing, with retirement in sight for many.

The view that 'bigger is better' is, of course, simplistic. The popular image of a 'poor' practice comprises an elderly single-handed doctor, in unattractive premises, providing limited availability of care. The main criticisms surrounding such practices is that they are unresponsive to change, for example resisting appointments systems and computers (although these are not necessarily markers for the quality of medicine practised). In other words, small practices may be more fragile organisations but poor doctors may be found in any practice. The clinical director of the Wolverhampton project, as GP tutor, concluded that a number of good single-handed GPs were feeling beleaguered: trying to run a business was too much for them. A resourceful management, taking over the organisation but re-employing the doctor, seemed to be one way of reducing early retirements and retaining skills.

More boldly, setting up a salaried option might improve recruitment of younger doctors who are reluctant to be tied into partnerships. The same scheme could use limited 'new' monies for PMS to launch new practices. Such a provider could have been 'stand alone' or part of an NHS trust. A further early ambition was to take over single-handed vacancies as they arose, though this has not occurred. Later, the scheme was asked to 'parachute' into struggling practices doctors who would either take them over or temporarily provide medical support. The intention was to provide the benefits of single-handed practice (continuity and personal care) with those of group practice (better management, flexibility, guaranteed holidays, study leave and sick pay). The package was to encourage doctors to join, stay, and enjoy their job.

The management and structure that evolved

Ultimately, the provider had to be the community trust because of the financial risk involved. The scheme in Wolverhampton currently has ten GPs, with a turnover of more than £1m. The trust drew the scheme into its higher management, which allowed cross fertilisation between general practice and other trust responsibilities such as district nursing and children's services.

We began with five existing patient lists (four were single handed and one doctor had left an unhappy partnership) and set up four new ones with pump-priming money. Two doctors are employed as extra GPs for other projects, including the running of failing practices. Practices are largely covered by the same doctors all the time (i.e. they have personal lists), though the GPs have to cross-cover for one another's absence. Income to support the scheme comes from a number of sources:

- Former practices bring the gross income they used to receive as GMS GPs.
- New practices bring in new money, at least for three years, until 'viable', which means a list of 2000 or so. We benefit from being better at claiming practice staff budgets, improvement grants and other GMS income streams. Again, this was negotiated with the health authority.
- We keep private income from medical reports, cremation certificates, etc., that doctors generate in working hours.
- We supply doctors to trusts, PCGs and other GPs at a fee, when we have the surplus capacity.
- We take on special projects such as occupational health and winter pressures work, again locally agreed.

The main costs over and above the running costs of nine practices are the manager, her assistant (both full time) and the clinical director (£7500 pa). This allows us to maintain financial balance without being more expensive to the health authority than a GMS doctor would be.

The salary schemes: terms and conditions

Most interest has been shown in our scheme as a model for employing salaried GPs, though it is more unusual for a number of other reasons. Primary care already has many doctors working for a salary: assistants are usually salaried; 'retainer scheme' doctors and registrars are salaried (with allowances); and the wisest arrangement for GPs considering a partnership is some kind of salaried system during the first few months of mutual assessment. Larger partnerships will usually have a business leader and, in contrast, it is common to find doctors in a profit-sharing scheme in which they play little active part. While not actually salaried, such doctors behave as such, willingly or through lack of interest, delegating their technical business responsibilities to the business partner. Salaries involve less advantageous tax rules but the net loss is not as great as many GPs think.

From the Wolverhampton scheme's point of view, a salary does allow a clear line of accountability and motivation. It clarifies the relationship between the doctor and the contract holder (the trust), and minimises conflicts of interest. Pay is the equivalent to a basic consultant salary after three years, plus GP seniority payments scale, travel and all expenses (See Tables 3.1 and 3.2)

Table 3.1 General practitioner salary scale

Basic consultant grade (NHS)			£48,905
General practitioners without principal experience	Year 1	80%	£39,126
	Year 2	90%	£44,016
	Year 3	95%	£46,461
	Year 4	100%	£48,905
GP seniority pay		after 6 years	£530 pa
		after 13 years	£2,805 pa
		after 19 years	£5,980 pa
		after 25 years	£7,275 pa
Expenses:		You should incur no personal expenses in this post Medical defence is covered under trust policies Mobile telephone and all medical kit supplied Travel allowance – £150 per month.	

Table 3.2 Wolverhampton Health Care NHS Trust person specification

	Essential	*Desirable*	*Method of assessment*
Educational/ qualifications	MB MS or equivalent. Must be approved to work as a GP by the JCPTGP. GMC Registration.	MRCGP	Application form and certificate to be shown at interview.
Experience	Recent experience in UK general practice (registrar or other). Prescribing in general practice.	Further experience relevant to general practice. Locum experience. Clinical support. Supervision.	Application form and interview.

continued

Table 3.2 *continued*

	Essential	*Desirable*	*Method of assessment*
Skills and abilities	The ability to communicate effectively. Patient focused.	Experience of working within the following clinical areas: • asthma • diabetes • family planning • minor surgery • child health surveillance • screening clinics • basic computer literacy • skills • teaching skills.	Application form and interview.
Other requirements	Evidence of and a commitment to continuing professional development. Commitment to confidentiality. Flexibility to meet the needs of the pilot and SE PCG. Self-motivated.	A sense of humour.	Application form and interview.

Pension

GPs joining the scheme who have not been principals before (e.g. having completed a vocational training scheme), join the NHS pension scheme at 'officer' status as any hospital doctor would. This gives a final pension based on final salary. GMS GPs transferring to PMS retain for the life of the pilot – initially three years, then extended – the same pension rights they had under their old contract; this calculates pensions differently, using lifetime earnings adjusted for inflation. The latter system has some advantages for GPs who have been in that role for most of their working lives. Doctors who become GPs later in their careers, or who never were GMS doctors, are often better off in the officer scheme, but the computation is complex and there is room for controversy – often 'exploited' by the BMA and others! Therefore, we arranged independent advice for all doctors joining our scheme but have not 'topped up' any doctor's pension.

Contract arrangements with staff

The rules for transferring staff are established in law, as the Transfer of Undertakings (Protection of Employment) regulations (TUPE). This has to be adhered to carefully. GPs do not have to stay within the Whitely Council NHS pay scales and we had some tricky adjustments to make when staff were moved. A trust can support staff development and training more effectively than small practices can. This is especially the case with the nursing staff who have become closer to, though not integrated with, the district nurses than any of the regular GMS practice nurses.

Recruitment

A major purpose of the Wolverhampton scheme has been to aid recruitment. The trust had a reasonable response to the first advertisement – for one vacancy in 1998. Six people were interviewed and five were considered appointable. The second wave created three further vacancies and the advertisement received more than 40 expressions of interest. Nine applicants were interviewed and most were appointable. At the time, a large number of PMS schemes were looking for doctors. GPs straight off vocational training schemes did not seem to want this work; however, in retrospect, our literature might have seemed off-putting to such doctors and we learned from this.

One doctor, employed by us but not with her own practice, is leaving to become a GMS partner in a local practice and, from the city's point of view, this is a success.

The GPs' responsibilities

All our GPs run their own practices, offering continuity of care for their patients and working with the small team at their site. They do standard surgeries of two or two-and-a-half hours twice a day, with visits and other commitments in between. They have to be available for their patients whenever the out-of-hours co-op is not covering them, which is from 7 a.m. to 7 p.m., except for a weekly half day from 1 p.m. Saturdays are not usually worked. List sizes are between 1700 and 2200.

It is not the clinical director's role to dictate how medical care should be given by an individual doctor. We do not dictate appointment length, but holidays have to be negotiated, as does any alteration in availability. Staff appointments are made by the manager, not the doctor. The premises are run by the trust but, as with non-clinical staff, the doctors' views are considered too (we hope).

Managing doctors and the clinical director

All trusts have a medical director who will vary in how much he or she imposes on the consultants; managing GPs presents similar challenges. The bottom line is that patients need seeing efficiently (the manager's job) and effectively (the GPs' job, with help and supervision). To achieve the former, a certain authority over the doctor is needed. All practices provide at least four hours booked surgeries a day, with sufficient numbers of 'urgent' slots. The GP is not able unilaterally to change this and can alter provision only after discussion with management.

All doctors have a duty to keep up to date, and there is positive encouragement to do this from the trust. Regular dialogue about personal development is supposed to take place. The written contract with the trust would form the basis of any disciplinary issue. Complaints are dealt with primarily by the manager and clinical director rather than by employed clinicians.

Do they work well?

A common question raised by other doctors is whether GPs on a salary work as well as profit-sharing doctors. This is a complex issue, since it presupposes we want doctors to work like GMS GPs when the latter's contracts may sometimes reward profitable rather than effective work. We are all aware of doctors who do not pull their weight and, conversely and more commonly, doctors who overwork through dedication to their patients. Salaried doctors reflect the same spread of attitudes, but at least we have a mechanism for performance managing the less motivated.

Holidays, study time, perks

Our scheme tries to allow for 'guilt-free' holidays and study time in reasonable measure, akin to Whitley Council entitlements. There are constraints in that cross-cover means holidays have to be negotiated and we cannot have too many doctors away at one time.

GPs are provided with everything they want, including a lease car, should they want one. Perks are few (see Box 3.1), but we do not forbid doctors earning money out of our hours so long as it does not affect performance.

Box 3.1 THE COST OF MOTORING FOR GPS

GPs feel a major perk of Schedule D self-employed taxation status is tax-deductible motoring. Including capital allowances and all expenses, a car might cost £4000 a year to run in Wolverhampton. In the old days, GPs used to claim 90 per cent of this as practice expense but most inspectors are not convinced by this, so let us assume 75 per cent, or £3000, is allowable. At 40 per cent tax rate this equates to £1200 a year relief. We give our doctors £150 a month for a car, which is taxable – a net payment of £90.

Appraisals and clinical governance

Doctors in our scheme are expected to engage in clinical governance activities. The local PCG clinical governance mechanisms apply to the Wolverhampton salaried doctors as they do to GMS principals. However, some aspects of clinical governance are best delegated back to management (such as health and safety issues and risk management) and others the managers assist with (such as staff support with audit and the provision of protected time for critical event discussions).

PMS doctors, like all doctors, have to keep up to date. Up to 30 hours of continuing professional development (CPD) is paid for GMS GPs, but the salaried scheme does not receive or pass on extra income for this obligation. The GP is expected to do much more than 30 hours and to keep a portfolio to prove it; the advent of Personal Learning Plans to advise which areas of CPD to concentrate on help with this. An annual appraisal scheme is in place but has proved difficult to implement so far, partly because of the clinical director's commitments. This will have a higher priority henceforth.

If a staff member, including a doctor, falls ill, the general manager has to arrange cover for the work that needs doing. This is the sort of practice 'hassle' GPs join the scheme to escape. Experience tells us that complaints are best handled by the trust complaints procedure, rather than by the doctor at the practice. Legal indemnity is covered by the trust. However, the role of a clinical director is to be supportive, and to date there have been no disciplinary problems.

Size of organisation

The Wolverhampton scheme of nine practices is viable, but we feel it has reached the point where further economies of scale would be small. There are about 50 employees and that, as well as being a part of a trust, contributes to a sense of remoteness of management from the front line. Team working should be at practice level, though the GPs also meet fortnightly as a team.

Relationship with other GPs

GPs feel they are being forced by the Government to work harder for less, and high-profile schemes like ours generate anxiety. Our LMC was initially neutral about us, but many individuals were against the idea and said so. After three years, we have proved to be more of a support than a threat to the local GP community, and are accepted as part of the health community. The prime reason for this is our determination to remain voluntary and to support independent contractor status where that works best.

Conclusion

Independent contractor status works less well in inner cities and for doctors who do not enjoy business partnerships. The poor quality of primary care in many urban areas demands new ways of working. A scheme like ours is one model of externally managed care using salaries, and has addressed some issues (recruitment and retention) better than others (clinical governance and premises management). A sizeable cohort of excellent GPs prefers a salary and it is good to offer this option. A national scheme standardising pay and conditions would help to form a basis for this in other areas. But, for many parts of the country, GMS provides the best deal for the community and is unlikely to be dismantled while it does.

Chapter 4

Improving waiting and access in the NHS – treating the cause

James Kingsland

KEY POINTS

This practice in Wallasey has used PMS Plus to generate significant efficiency gains. The experience has helped sustain high morale at a time of major change.

Introduction

St Hilary Brow Group Practice serves a population of 5500 in the semi-urban area of Wallasey, situated on the north-east tip of the Wirral peninsula. The practice had been fundholding since 1992 but, by 1996, was looking for a new direction focusing on the provision of general practice rather than the ability to purchase secondary care services. Following an intensive preparatory period, the practice applied to be a first wave PMS pilot. The practice took the 'leap of faith', not only by resigning from fundholding a year early, but also by resigning from the Part II Medical List of Wirral Health Authority to negotiate a local service agreement over a three-year pilot period.

PMS pilots were seen as a means to enhance and expand the provision of primary care services at practice level, to develop more flexible working relationships between the primary health care professionals based at the practice, and to focus clinical efforts on patient needs rather than the activities directed by the national GMS contract.

Background

St Hilary Brow Group Practice is known for innovation. In each of the three years from 1996 to 1998, the National Association of Fundholding

Practices recognised its achievements with one of their prestigious innovation awards. Chartermark has also highly commended the practice on two separate occasions for its patient services. The practice believes that to provide high-quality, accessible primary care, services need to be developed within practice, in particular by increasing the number and range of human resources available. The PMS pilot was seen as an opportunity to shift a good deal of work currently carried out in hospital to the practice. The aim was to redefine the primary care 'package', reduce waiting lists and catalyse hospitals to reconsider how best to deploy specialist clinical staff.

Research by the practice has shown that the majority of patients seen as follow-up outpatients do not need to be seen in hospital. Furthermore, with more services within the practice, a substantial number of new referrals could be avoided.

The motivation behind this is simple. The primary care setting offers:

- greater continuity of care
- easier accessibility
- a more appropriate, co-ordinated, follow-up regime
- potentially lower costs
- fewer GP/hospital transactions, with less effort and less cost
- greater responsiveness to patients, with increased satisfaction.

There are also a number of benefits from the hospital point of view:

- waiting times can be reduced
- consultants are free to consult
- hospitals have the chance to increase productivity without investing in additional clinical staff
- the training of junior doctors in general practice can be broadened.

The practice reviewed a three-month sample of hospital discharge letters and found that 75 per cent of follow-up appointments required only low technology support and were of low complexity. Only 25 per cent required special diagnostics or the opinion of a consultant or senior member of the junior staff. Annually, this 75 per cent amounts to some

1000 follow-up consultations. The analysis also suggested that about 200 new attendances could have been avoided had an alternative service been available. This activity was costed by the health authority (discussed below). There was also the opportunity to reduce some inpatient costs, both in terms of procedures performed and 'patient bed days'.

The practice appointed a project manager from within the existing practice team resources to co-ordinate the project and carry out the hospital and patient liaison required for the project.

Pilot aims and objectives

The pilot aimed to focus on disease management provided by a dedicated practice-based primary health care team.

As a pilot, the partnership operated a 'PMS Plus' practice-based contract and offered a new salaried position for a general practitioner. Two objectives were identified: to provide the community with a seamless provision of care that was responsive to the registered population's needs; and to plan the services more effectively across both primary and secondary care (thereby improving accessibility and providing greater continuity of care for patients). This was to be achieved by facilitating the move of caseloads of low complexity (requiring low-technology care) from secondary care back to primary care. This would allow both primary and secondary care professionals to use their skills more appropriately.

To achieve this, an increase in the capacity and skill mix of the primary health care team was required, as were more flexible employment opportunities. This team could then deliver primary care and develop clinical care pathways, reducing the range and volume of primary care-type procedures performed in a secondary care setting. It was expected that the number of referrals of low-complexity patients to acute facilities would reduce, as would the number of follow-up outpatient appointments. As a consequence, a reduction of hospital waiting lists was anticipated.

The primary care team

The primary care team assembled to deliver PMS at the practice is as follows:

- Three-and-a-half whole time equivalent GPs (using the GMS definition) delivering between them the equivalent of 24 half-day sessions per week. This in effect meant there are two GPs in the practice, all day, every day.
- A full-time GP registrar is usually in post, together with a further doctor on the 'retainer scheme'. While these are educational posts, this provides the equivalent of a further GP on a daily basis.
- Three practice-employed nurses with varying skills and experience (1.5 whole time equivalent).
- One half-day counselling session in the practice per week.
- One whole time equivalent health visitor and dedicated practice-attached district nursing team.

During the preparatory period, the practice gained the agreement of the health authority and local community trust to the secondment of other health care professionals on a sessional basis, commensurate with the practice's current referral rate. The following staff were seconded to the practice for the duration of the pilot:

- a dietician for two half-day sessions per month
- an occupational therapist for one half-day session per week
- a community psychiatric nurse for two practice-based sessions per week
- a clinical psychologist for between one and two half-day sessions per month.

To complete the team and to meet the pilot's objectives, further personnel requirements were identified:

- a three-quarter whole time equivalent general practitioner
- a half whole time equivalent practice nurse
- additional physiotherapy sessions
- a nurse clinician to lead on a range of mental health projects and cancer service initiatives
- additional counselling services.

To facilitate the funding of these additional posts, the preparatory period before the pilot went live was used to assess the scope for transferring patients currently under hospital care back to the practice for follow-up. In addition, the potential for reducing new referrals to hospital through practice-based services and direct access to high-technology investigations was assessed.

The practice was already a relatively low user of hospital services (indeed, one of the lowest referrers to hospital in Wirral). However, the practice believed that this referral and follow-up rate could be reduced further if extra funding was made available to the primary care team. This estimated reduction of hospital contacts was costed (at about £50,000) by the health authority and the local acute trust, and this resource was made available to the practice by the health authority (from growth) as a 'plus' element to their PMS contract. The practice decided to use this money to employ a 0.75 WTE salaried GP, to fund some extra-practice nursing hours, and to pay the community trust for practice-based physiotherapy sessions. The latter would deal with a range of musculo-skeletal, chronic chest and female urinary incontinence problems.

A nurse clinician from the community trust with expertise in mental health and palliative care was also seconded to the practice at no cost to examine the potential to improve community mental health services within the practice. Finally, the practice decided to use some of its own funds and staffing budget to employ an extra counsellor to provide an additional two sessions a week. The team was now in place and the practice was charged by its commissioner to demonstrate a significant shift of patients from hospital back into primary care.

Developing the model and consultation

Practice-based patient management would be extended in four ways:

- reduction in referral rates to all specialties
- early discharge of patients from follow-up in hospital outpatient departments
- reduction in outpatient contacts for patients by directly accessing a range of high-technology procedures not normally available to GPs

and also directly admitting patients to operating lists for certain agreed diagnostic procedures, e.g. gastroscopy, colonoscopy, hysteroscopy, cystoscopy

- making efficient use of community health care professionals not normally practice-attached to improve efficiency and to reduce waiting times for those services, consequently reducing the need for referral outside the practice.

A system diagram was developed to show clearly to patients how they would be recalled from hospital (see Figure 4.1). This was important in ensuring that patients fully understood the pilot's objectives and in securing their agreement to practice-based management.

During the preparatory period, the practice members consulted widely about their ideas, particularly to see if their patients would welcome this type of service. The practice had already set up a Patient Advisory Panel, and used this as a forum to debate service development at the practice. This panel carried out an extensive survey of patient opinion, which showed that a large majority (95 per cent) welcomed the proposal.

The senior partner in the practice, together with the chief executive of the health authority, visited the local acute trust board and council to explain the pilot. In addition, doctors at the practice made contact with every clinical directorate to discuss the pilot's ambitions and the clinical processes it would employ.

Results and evaluation

The evaluation of the project became a joint effort between the practice, the health authority and the acute trust. This was supplemented by an external evaluation of the project, carried out by the Department of Clinical Psychology at the University of Liverpool. This latter evaluation focused on how well the integrated practice team worked together and patients' satisfaction with the service. It also commented on the sustainability, transferability and added value of the project to the local health economy and how easily it could be reproduced.

Figure 4.1 The process of patient recall from hospital outpatient department

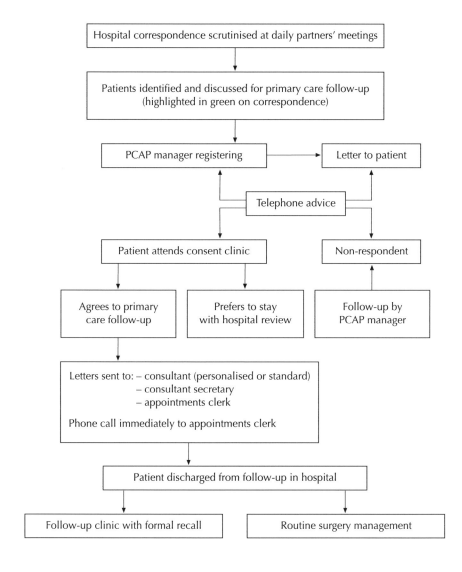

A sample of 200 responses from patients who had been contacted to transfer their routine care back to practice showed that 98 per cent preferred to come to surgery for follow-up.

The most frequent reasons given for this preference were:

- consistency
- reduced waiting time
- friendly and more familiar surroundings
- better communication
- local, more accessible centre for health care.

The scheme had also been met with enthusiasm by hospital secretaries and appointment clerks, who were delighted to be able to 'free up' appointments for reallocation. If extended over the whole health authority, this model could have a significant impact on the availability of appointments and waiting list times in hospital.

Table 4.1 below provides data on the comparative referral rates between the practice, the PCG and the health authority for all attendances in the outpatients of the local acute trust. These figures confirm that, though St Hilary Brow was historically a low-referring practice when compared with the PCG and health authority average, attendances were reduced further in the first pilot year.

Table 4.1 Comparison of referral rates: practice, PCG, health authority

Acute trust outpatients – all attendances
Rate per 1000 outpatients – age standardised and indexed (HA = 1) for all specialties

	Practice	*PCG*	*Health authority*
Preparatory year	0.64	0.84	1.0
Pilot year 1	0.42	0.77	1.0
(PCG data included practice)			

Source: Wirral Health Authority

Table 4.2 demonstrates the use of the acute trust's outpatient department for first attendance compared with that of the PCG and health authority. During the preparatory year, the comparative rate of referral from the practice was half that of the health authority. However, during the first year of the pilot, this rate fell to less than 30 per cent of the health authority average, showing that a further reduction in referral rate was achievable given appropriate resources at practice level. The PCG average also fell over the same time period compared to the health authority average, but the pilot reduction outstripped this despite starting from a lower base. These figures have been sustained, but not reduced further, over the subsequent two years of the pilot. The scope for further reduction was minimal and would not have been clinically appropriate.

Table 4.2 Comparison of outpatient usage: practice, PCG, health authority

Acute trust outpatients – first attendance
Rate per 1000 outpatients – age standardised and indexed (HA = 1) for all specialties

	Practice	PCG	Health authority
Preparatory year	0.54	0.85	1.0
Pilot year 1	0.29	0.78	1.0
(PCG data included practice)			

Source: Wirral Health Authority

It is important to note that low referrals and a low use of hospital services do not always equate with quality and best practice. However, the range of practice-based services available at St Hilary Brow and, as a consequence, the range of therapeutic interventions, suggest that patients are being managed more extensively in the community. Ongoing qualitative audit confirms this.

Extending the management of patients in primary care and using hospital services less for primary care work is clinically effective and gives great value for money to the NHS. This significantly improves primary care services, professional development and morale in those primary carers providing them.

In the first year of the pilot, the efficiency savings made by the practice due to reduced hospital activity was approximately £60,000. As a result of an initial investment by Wirral Health Authority of £50,000 in the PMS Plus contract, there was a saving of approximately £10,000.

This demonstrates that this type of investment is cost-effective (if the primary care service is well managed). If extrapolated across the health authority, this could realise a saving of 50 times this amount, in addition to a potentially significant reduction in hospital waiting times.

It is also important to note that the activity data has been collected from the main acute trust provider. The practice also uses services in other hospitals in Merseyside, but to a lesser extent. This activity has not been reconciled with the health authority, but Tables 4.3 and 4.4 below show the practice's data on its recall activity and reduction in hospital referrals in the first year. In addition to the reduction in referrals and outpatient contacts, 20 patients received direct radiological investigation in that year, using procedures that previously would have required an initial referral to a consultant. A further 62 patients were listed for direct endoscopy assessment and 31 admitted directly onto a consultant surgeon's operating list without prior outpatient assessment. An increase in minor surgery activity in practice further reduced the need for referral to hospital. The final reduction in total outpatient appointments for the practice in the first year was 994, and for the local acute trust the reduction was 337. Both these figures were confirmed by the health authority.

Table 4.3 Outpatient recalls – year 1

Appointments (identified)	497
Number thought to be inappropriate for recall following team meeting	54
Patient letters sent	443
Patients followed up in surgery (discharged from hospital)	367 (83%)
Patients who preferred to stay in outpatient department	32 (7%)
Non-respondents	44 (10%)

Table 4.4 New patient referrals – all specialties

Pre-pilot years	1996/7	671
	1997/8	614
Pilot year	1998/9	366

Downward trends were found in all specialties

Conclusion

The new system of care was well received by patients. This finding was confirmed by the patient advisory panel, which carried out interviews with patients, and by the University of Liverpool, which carried out an independent evaluation commissioned by the health authority.

The expansion of primary care services has been a cost-effective investment by the commissioner. A 'triple whammy' in terms of cost-effectiveness has been observed in the direct savings achieved by the practice, through the freeing-up of hospital appointments, and through greater responsiveness (leading to increased patient satisfaction). If adopted more widely, this model of delivering services could reduce waiting times for hospital services and improve access. Though a relatively small practice, St Hilary Brow achieved a reduction of 994 outpatient contacts in its first year. If this figure were extrapolated to a health authority, or indeed to a national level, the impact on the health service could be enormous.

This suggests that there is the potential to make savings in the local health economy budget. While some local sceptics have questioned whether a saving of £10,000 is really that significant, it is worth pointing out that the practice was already working effectively before the pilot started. For less-efficient practices, with much larger registered populations, the potential for savings would be much greater. Importantly, morale has been sustained in the practice at a high level, and efficient working between primary health care professionals has been reported by the independent evaluation team.

Chapter 5

Nurse-led general practice – the implications of nurse-led practice for nurses, doctors and patients

Catherine Baraniak and Lance Gardner

KEY POINTS

Nurses can build and lead primary health care teams. Patients appreciate the care they receive but this has sometimes been in spite of rather than because of the support of other local providers.

Introduction

The NHS (Primary Care) Act 1997 provided an opportunity for individuals other than GPs to contract to provide primary medical care for patients. Several community trust-led proposals appeared from around the country suggesting that nurses should have a greater role in delivering patient care. However, two proposals, one from Derby and one from Salford, were submitted by individual nurses. In these proposals, a nurse would enter into an agreement with the local health authority to provide medical services as an independent contractor. The nurse would be self-employed and would personally employ the other members of a team, tailored to meet the needs of the patient community.

The two nurse leads – Catherine Baraniak in Derby and Lance Gardner in Salford – set out to identify whether there would be any benefits to patients, staff and the wider NHS in using a nurse-led model of providing care. In this model, a nurse rather than a GP acts as the first point of contact for the patient. Moreover, nurse-led care does not necessarily follow the traditional 'biomedical' model of care. The biomedical model approaches the presenting problem from an illness perspective, with the GP recommending action, treatment or referral; the nurse-led model, on the other hand, suggests that, as many of the problems presenting in surgeries are not medically oriented, someone other than a GP is capable of deciding how patients' needs can be met. Of course, a nurse can also work using a biomedical approach and, in a nurse-led setting, frequently does.

The nurse-led models being developed in Salford and Derby aim to utilise as wide a body of professionals as possible to meet the needs of their communities, to ensure that patients' concerns are addressed by the most appropriate person to help them. The hope is that patients will begin to lose the notion that they must have an illness of some sort before they can be seen in the surgery, thereby enabling them to talk about other more pressing needs that may not be of a medical nature.

The conception of nurse-led and GP-led practice as two ends of a continuum can be challenged. While the outcomes of national and local evaluations of first wave PMS pilots are still awaited, our experience is that neither a solely GP-led model nor a solely nurse-led model of care provision can be claimed to be the best way of providing services for patients. We have concluded that a team approach to care, utilising the skills and strengths of all team members, is the most appropriate way to meet the diversity of patient need. We have used the term 'nurse-led care' throughout this chapter. However, by this we mean a multidisciplinary approach within which nurses are able to use their skills to the full. The 'nurse-led' label is used to emphasise an equality between professionals and to challenge the often-automatic assumption that doctors are the 'natural' leaders of primary care.

What is nurse-led primary care?

The term 'nurse-led' is currently used in a variety of settings, and suggests a continuum of practice ranging from the nurse having delegated authority to make decisions regarding patient care at one end of the spectrum, to being responsible for all care provided (including the clinical assessment, treatment and management of patients undifferentiated by need) at the other. As nurses' responsibility for greater degrees of patient care increases, so too does their management of the resources to provide such care. Both employed and self-employed nurses can provide nurse-led care, as the nurse-led element depends on the decision-making autonomy of the nurse and not the nurse's employment status. Nurse-led primary care reflects a model of service in which nurses have a higher profile in providing care for patients, based on their own assessment of the patient's needs. Their decisions will be based on their level of skill and ability, and their interpretation of their scope of practice. Decision-making may be supported by practice protocols or guidelines, or by parameters set by their employers. In the case of practice nurses, this employer would normally be the GP.

For the two PMS pilots being considered in this chapter, nurse-led primary care encompasses all of the above, but it also includes responsibility for the physical provision of care services, provided by the most appropriately skilled people. The two nurses hold service agreements with their respective health authorities, and take responsibility for providing these services by putting in place the infrastructure and multidisciplinary team required to address the community's needs.

A brief overview of the two pilots is provided in Boxes 5.1 and 5.2.

Nurse-led practice can impact significantly on job satisfaction, not just for those nurses working as independent contractors but also for those working within the practice teams.[1] In-house observations at the Meadowfields Practice suggest that the GP enjoys a high level of job satisfaction. This stems from the freedom to pursue other clinical interests and the opportunity to see patients with significant medical problems, as opposed to routine or minor issues. The ethos of nurse-led primary care – that the patient should be seen by the most appropriate person – emphasises the decision-making and care-giving role of every team member. We believe that the skills and abilities of all are used to the full (and, in the interests of efficiency, are used appropriately), generating an understanding and appreciation of each team member's role, and leading to levels of morale and satisfaction seldom seen in the health service. It is important to emphasise that nurse-led practice does not seek to replace the role of the GP but to ensure that it is carried out with maximum effectiveness.

Box 5.1 The Meadowfields Practice, Chellaston, Derby

The Meadowfields Practice opened on 24 August 1998. It is a new practice, set on the outskirts of Derby in an area of substantial new housing development with a mixed socio-economic structure. It is unlikely that difficulties would be experienced in recruiting a traditional general practitioner. The practice opened with a list of 500 patients, grew to 2000 patients by the end of the second year, stood at 2500 patients at the beginning of 2001, and continues to grow. The practice is open to patients for 53 hours per week, offering early morning and late night services. All morning sessions operate on a drop-in basis. There are eight members of the practice team, including clerical and administrative staff. The community trust provides community nursing services. Although patients are given the choice of who they consult, they are encouraged to see the nurse as their first point of contact.

Box 5.2 The Daruzzaman Care Centre, Salford, Manchester

The Daruzzaman Care Centre opened on 1 April 1998 in Salford, an inner city area with high levels of deprivation and need. The physical and economic environment of inner city and socially deprived areas has a significant impact on the health needs of local communities. A nurse-led model was proposed, which emphasised holistic care and 'normalisation'. This was deemed to be more appropriate in meeting specific local needs than a more traditional biomedical model of care. The former GP, Dr Daruzzaman, died in post, leaving a vacant list that was adopted in its entirety by the new PMS pilot. There are 18 members of the practice team, with the practice nurse, district nurses and health visitor being employed by the local community trust. Patients can choose to see a GP or a nurse.

However, despite high levels of job satisfaction evident in both practices, the two pilots have experienced similar challenges in the implementation of their pilots. In particular, certain NHS policies, procedures and legislative issues have all put obstacles in the way of providing services for patients. It is the purpose of a pilot to uncover such issues. However, if the model of care provision is to be replicated elsewhere, these issues need to be resolved to prevent frustration and stunted progress among those that follow on in the future.

Particular challenges experienced by the nurse-led pilots have included:

- a lack of a nationally recognised qualification for nurses taking on extended nursing roles
- the absence of adequate prescribing rights and access to the British National Formulary for nurses
- the responsibility for the prescribing budget, which is drawn upon by the GPs
- the absence of authority to sign sickness certificates and other paperwork relating to welfare benefits
- the lack of recognition of the nurse as the 'attending physician' prior to a patient's death and lack of authority to sign a death certificate
- securing referral rights to secondary care and other agencies
- obtaining liability insurance for self-employed nurses
- the registration of patients with GPs who are employed by nurses
- the allocation of resources using an historical GMS baseline.

The rest of this chapter examines these issues in more depth and considers their implications from the standpoint of the nursing profession, the medical profession and patients themselves.

Implications of 'nurse-led' practice for the nursing profession

Extension of nursing skills

Nurses in primary care have been the first point of contact for some patients for many years. However, this approach has been formalised and extended within our pilots, with the result that nurses are now exposed to a much higher degree of first contact care. Although patients are given the choice of whether they see a GP or a nurse (and, in the Meadowfields Practice, the nurse manages approximately 50 to 65 per cent of patients with little reference to the GP), many of the patients who choose to see the GP present with problems that could in fact be managed by the nurse. The nurse-led model of care requires a huge increase in competence for nurses based on clinical expertise, clinical judgement and autonomous practice. While the pilot nurses are not aiming to be 'mini-doctors', they need a significantly higher level of clinical education and skill development than they would in a 'traditional' primary care nursing role. This has proved difficult to find within the current nursing establishment. In contrast, GP registrar schemes offer a system of ongoing education that could address this need. The establishment from scratch of a radically different model of care requires the nurse leads to work in an environment of uncertainty, and means that the pilots are 'breaking the mould' virtually every day.

Traditionally, nurses have enjoyed the safety of supervised practice and the use of protocols or policies. However, in nurse-led pilots this has simply not proved possible. Furthermore, there are currently few education programmes that prepare nurses to provide care at this level of practice with such degrees of uncertainty. Educational establishments need to begin encouraging nurses to think beyond their more traditional ways of working. Clinical skills must also be underpinned by an academic standing that enables nurses to work as equals with other professionals, particularly doctors, not all of whom support extended nursing roles.

Clinical skills, however, make up only a small component of the wide range of skills required to help patients in general practice. A health needs assessment at the Meadowfields Practice demonstrated that a very high proportion of patients attended the surgery with problems that needed neither medical nor nursing care, but did so because they did not know where else to go for help. At the Daruzzaman Care Centre, the number of patients in this socially deprived population presenting without medical needs was even higher. Both nurse leads act as 'signposts' to other services and this is a crucial element of their role. Consequently, strong links have been made with a wide range of agencies who may offer more appropriate support than those in primary care, such as Victim Support, Relate, social services, the probation service and alcohol/drug rehabilitation schemes.

Prescribing

Prescribing has proved a significant issue for both pilots. 'Specialist–generalist' nurses, such as PMS pilot nurse leads, need access to the whole drug formulary (rather than the extremely limited formulary currently allowed under the current nurse prescribing regulations). Furthermore, the independent nurse contractor must take responsibility for the pilot's drug budget but has little effective control over how their GP employees spend it.

A study of nurse prescribing trends at the Meadowfields Practice during the first year of the pilot suggested that, had the nurses been able to prescribe, they would have accessed most areas of the formulary. Other studies of nurse prescribing over recent years have come to the same conclusions.[2] The development of patient group directions (locally agreed protocols regulating the supply of prescribed medicines by non-medical professionals) may go some way to resolving this issue, but it would be more appropriate for nurses to be able to prescribe based on their interpretation of clinical findings, supported by the law, and held accountable by their own signature on the prescription.

Sections of the GP community may well be anxious, as they contemplate nurses being let loose with a prescribing pad, about both cost and patient safety. But why should nurses act immoderately? They will be aware of their responsibility for spending part of the local drug budget as well as their responsibility for their own actions, the safety of the patient and their legal responsibility once their signature is on the prescription. For nurse-led pilots to be truly effective, the current nurses' formulary must be extended beyond such items as headlice lotions and laxatives.

Currently, the nurses of the Meadowfields Practice are not qualified nurse prescribers. In the practice setting, those prescriptions generated by the nurse must be signed by the GP. There is a strong element of trust that has developed between the GP and the nurse regarding the choice and suitability of drugs to be prescribed, based on familiarity with each others' prescribing patterns and practice policies. However, this is not a suitable basis for a local prescribing policy as it perpetuates the inadequacy of the current system – it leaves the GP exposed and liable for prescribing errors made by the nurse and it takes up additional time in surgery for doctor, nurse and patient. The nurses involved in the first wave of PMS pilots hoped that the new Health and Social Care Act would offer suitably trained and experienced nurses the opportunity to prescribe. However, only limited measures will be taken to increase the number of prescription-only medicines that nurses may prescribe in accordance with the Medicines Control Agency.[3]

Certification

In addition to prescribing, several other regulatory obstacles exist to impede day-to-day working of the nurses in the pilots. It is not possible, for example, for a community nurse to sign a sickness certificate in order for patients to claim Social Security and Statutory Sick Pay. Hospital nurses, however, are able to issue these. It is assumed that a patient is ill and unable to attend work if he or she is in hospital, yet there is no assessment or decision-making element involved. Community nurses are able to assess the patient and determine capability for work, as well as gauge how long the patient should be off sick.

Similarly, nurses are not recognised as the 'attending physician' prior to a patient's death. Despite numerous visits by nurses to a dying patient, unless seen by a GP, the patient would be required to undergo a post-mortem examination to establish cause of death. This situation arose in Salford during the first year of the pilot and, as a consequence, the patient's family and the nurse lead were subject to undue stress and anxiety.

Referrals

The creation of good multidisciplinary working within nurse-led primary care teams has been successfully achieved in both pilots. However, developing relationships with secondary care consultants (particularly securing the right of nurses to make direct referrals) has been more problematic. In Salford, the nurse lead secured referral rights at the commencement of the pilot by writing to each consultant in the local acute trusts, engaging their support. In Derby, individual referrals were made to one consultant at a time, securing referral acceptance by 'earning a hearing' with each doctor. These referrals have been accepted, but agreed protocols need to be established if universal and permanent nurse referral rights are to be secured. This assumes, of course, that consultants and their trade union will be willing to collaborate.

Professional representation

Nurse-led practice has attracted a great deal of local and national interest – medical and nursing organisations, politicians and the media have all been keenly interested in the work and development of the pilots. Pilot nurse leaders have been placed in a position of professional leadership, but they themselves need support to carry out this role; individual nurse leaders have developed their own support networks both locally and nationally. However, no formally recognised structure exists that can be called upon.

In contrast, the BMA is able to offer support to GPs as they negotiate their PMS contracts (including advice on contracts, staffing, pay and the law). Notwithstanding constant encouragement from the Royal College of Nursing, no such tangible support exists for nurses. Even in relation to indemnity insurance with respect to the actions of employees of independent contractors, no packages are currently available for nurses. Independent contractor nurses have had to obtain insurance from medical insurance companies. If the Royal College of Nursing's vision of nurse-led practice is to be achieved, these practical issues must be addressed.

Implications for the medical profession

Salaried general practice

While the nurse-led pilots were not originally proposed to address the issue of GP recruitment and retention, a spin-off of both pilots has been the creation of a new and attractive employment option for some doctors. The roles created by the two pilots are unique and the doctors are working in new ways. At Meadowfields, surplus GP time (prior to the practice list reaching its current 2600) was used to provide cover for a project for homeless people for two sessions a week. This provided the GP with the opportunity to pursue an interest in the care of people with drug and alcohol addiction, and also provided valuable income for the practice. Being salaried has relieved the GP from administrative duties and out-of-hours commitments, and has ensured an appropriate distribution of the clinical workload and use of complementary clinical skills. However, if these types of posts are to be extended, support must be put in place for salaried PMS doctors to ensure they are paid correctly, receive ongoing education, and maintain and develop their clinical skills. These issues are germane to all salaried GPs, whether working in a nurse-led practice or not, and lessons should be learned from the way in which many practice nurses have been treated by employers over the years.

Some ambiguities have arisen regarding the clinical responsibilities of the salaried GP in the Meadowfields pilot. The GP has salaried status, but maintains clinical responsibility for the patients on the list as they must, by law, be registered with him. However, the nurse lead of the pilot has had to take out additional employer's liability insurance to protect against a patient choosing to sue the employer rather than the GP in the event of a medical error. Further difficulties may arise for other organisations as a result of salaried status. For example, the local GP out-of-hours co-operative suggested that, as the salaried GP was not an independent contractor, the directors of the co-operative must assume responsibility for patients out of hours. Consequently, charges made by the co-operative to the Meadowfields pilot were significantly higher that those to other GP members. This created a heavy financial burden on the pilot. The solution was to identify a practice of independent GP principals that would assume responsibility for the Meadowfield's list out of hours. Consequently, fees have now been reduced to that for any other practice of a similar size.

Impact on primary care funding

There has been comment from many GPs suggesting that nurse-led practices receive funding above that of traditional GMS practices. This has not been the case. The Meadowfields Practice receives a budget based on the income generated by a single-handed GP with a list size of 2100 patients. Although the Meadowfields list exceeded 2000 patients during the second year of the pilot, the budget has not been enhanced to meet this higher capitation figure. In addition, the GP sees approximately 40 per cent of the number of patients seen in his previous GP principal post. Consequently, there is scope to increase registration and to manage a larger list than would be typical of a traditional single-handed GP practice. In Salford, much work has centred on community development. This activity does not attract a traditional item of service payment and is therefore unfunded. All community work has been undertaken within the fixed PMS budget.

Implications for patients

Patient satisfaction

Nurse-led pilots have also introduced a culture change for patients. Patients are far more likely to see a nurse than a doctor when visiting the surgery. It is important for both pilots that patients are comfortable with this change and that they accept it. Both pilots have reported high levels of patient satisfaction, with many patients quite happy to see a nurse and to see a nurse on a subsequent occasion without any reservations. The Salford practice has found that a significant proportion of patients do not really mind who sees them so long as someone can help with their problem.[4] Meadowfields has identified that the majority of patients have joined the practice as a result of a friend's or relative's recommendation, or that they have been 'attracted' to the nurse-led service.

Access

Both pilots ensure ease of access to services. The Salford pilot is open for 48 hours per week, offering open-access consultations for 33 of these hours. Meadowfields is open for 53 hours per week and offers a mixture of open access sessions and booked appointments. Patients are also able to choose which professional they see, and this includes a nurse or doctor, a district nurse, a health visitor, counsellor, community psychiatric nurse or any other member of the care team.

Patient involvement

Both pilots have been committed to developing a patient 'voice' and to encouraging patient involvement in the work of the practices. Patients have been key players in advising on the design of services and both practices have introduced structured patient access as a result (for example, a 7 a.m. start time and an 8 p.m. finish, together with Saturday opening and teenager-friendly surgeries). Health needs analysis work in both pilots has incorporated the views of patients and has identified them as expert in identifying the needs of the area. Health needs analysis carried out at Meadowfields incorporated the views of patients and others living locally. As a result, parenting sessions for families who may be isolated, afternoon coffee sessions for people new to the area, and family-friendly surroundings in the surgery, have been developed. The strong community emphasis of the practice is reflected by frequent coffee mornings, the regular newsletters posted to every household registered with the practice and the thriving patient participation group.

The Daruzzaman Care Centre has taken this one step further by becoming one of the three Commissioning for Well-Being projects in Manchester and Salford. These projects have developed a governing body along similar lines to that currently operating in schools with parent governors. The governing body manages a delegated budget on behalf of the local community with the intention of developing patient-centred services. They are in a position to effect real change for the local community.

Conclusion

The nurse-led model of care challenges several areas of traditional health care provision. While the term 'nurse-led' has been used since the inception of the pilots, it has become apparent that there is no need to elevate one profession above another. Instead, a team approach to problem solving and care planning offers the most comprehensive and appropriate use of skills. There is currently much discussion about working across traditional boundaries within the NHS, and between health and social care. This is a key theme of the NHS Plan. Our experience running nurse-led pilots suggests that there are a number of operational obstacles, which have been discussed above, that need to be overcome if this aspiration is to be made a reality.

The nurses and other staff in our PMS pilots have worked to overcome many of these issues. Some onlookers have gazed with wonder (if not alarm) at the temerity of the nurses and their teams as they challenge the *status quo*. Others have been excited by it and can see the benefits of trying out different models to find their strengths and weaknesses. Undoubtedly, some doctors have felt threatened, and have exhibited this by hostility towards the pilots and members of the practice teams (though many also admit to the need to change current arrangements).

Despite these tensions, both nurse leads have identified with many of the everyday problems faced by GPs. The problems of working within finite budgets and dealing with demands from patients, the health authority and the PCT have generated empathy across the nurse–GP divide. Both pilots have demonstrated a model that provides both high-quality primary care and excellent access. Both models are working within equitable budgets and are demonstrating improved job satisfaction for all those working in the pilots. The climate within primary care has changed in the last three years as organisations consider the arrival of PCG/Ts, with their different models of health care planning and different models of care delivery. There is a fear among the nurse-led pilots that PCTs will stifle the creativity of the practices and require them to conform to more traditional ways of working. Whether it is easier to convince a health authority of the merits of the pilots than it is a group of local GPs with whom you must work, and whose livelihoods may be affected as a consequence, only time will tell.

References

1   Chapple A, Sergison M. Challenging tradition. *Nursing Times* 1999; 95 (12): 32–3.
2   Mayes M. A study of prescribing patterns in the community. *Nursing Standard* 1996; 10 (29): 34–7.
3   Department of Health. *Patients to get quicker access to medicines.* Press release, 4 May 2001.
4   Chapple A, Rogers A, Macdonald W, Sergison M. Patients' perceptions of changing professional boundaries and the future of 'nurse-led' services. *Primary Health Care Research and Development* 2000; 1: 51–9.

Chapter 6

PMS Plus – developing a new organisation and extending services

Tim Richardson and Andrew Roscoe

KEY POINTS

The Integrated Care Partnership in Epsom has used PMS Plus to offer an extended range of practice-based services. They have imaginative plans to extend these to other practices in the locality, developing a new kind of primary care organisation in the process

Introduction

The Integrated Care Partnership (ICP) was created by the merger of three general practices in Epsom and Ewell in Surrey in April 1998. The fundamental reason for the merger was the preservation of the extended range of services the practices had developed individually for their local populations. The new ICP maintained its two historic sites

Figure 6.1 The Integrated Care Partnership PMS Plus Pilot

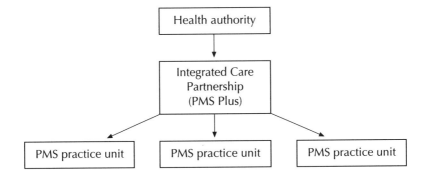

and continued to provide the full range of PMS services tailored to the needs of individuals. At the same time, PMS Plus was used as a vehicle to combine those extended services set up previously by the practices as GP fundholders and, later, by a total purchasing pilot. The creation of a locality-based organisation under PMS was therefore evolutionary and built on what had gone before. The ICP now serves a local population of 24,200 and includes 20 GPs (of whom 12 are partners), 12 nurses and 38 non-medical staff.

Providing extended in-house services

The three practices had built up a substantial range of extended 'in-house' services. These included:

- minor surgery
- physiotherapy
- dietetics
- ultrasound
- shared care outpatient specialist clinics.

They had also extended nurse provider roles and offered a range of nurse-led clinics, including those for diabetes, respiratory medicine and family planning. In addition, the practices had developed multi-agency, proactive care teams for complex care needs, such as for the elderly and patients suffering from neurological conditions.

By contracting to provide these services under PMS Plus, the practices ceased to function as health purchasers. Instead, the ICP shifted its role to become providers with direct service accountability to the health authority under a three-year contract (consequently, fundholding status was ended a year early as a condition of PMS Plus). The practices retained their total purchasing budget, which was 'top-sliced' by the health authority to resource the PMS Plus contract (see Box 6.1).

More unusually, one practice had co-developed and then taken over a day surgery hospital providing fully equipped specialist clinic facilities. These included a general and local anaesthetic-operating complex and X-ray and purpose-built physiotherapy facilities. It was and remains fully

---

Box 6.1 PMS PLUS SERVICES

- District nursing and health visiting (staff were seconded from the community trust to, and worked directly with and for, the practices).
- Direct access services, including physiotherapy, dietetics and near-site pathology, including anticoagulation care.
- Imaging, including plain X-ray, and on-site ultrasound (excluding antenatal).
- Shared care specialist clinics (supported by GPs and nurses undertaking follow-up care where appropriate).
- Surgical specialties include: ENT, orthopaedics, urology, general and plastic surgery, gynaecology (including a full colposcopy service), head and neck surgery, and ophthalmology.
- Medical specialties include: general medicine, diabetes, respiratory medicine, neurology, rheumatology, sports injuries, dermatology and care of the elderly.
- An open-access gastroscopy service.
- Elderly care, involving a nurse and GP clinical assistant working with our main acute provider hospital to facilitate discharge planning and co-ordination with community and social care.
- GP-managed cottage hospital beds.
- A GP minor surgery service.

---

accredited by the local health authority under the 1984 Nursing Homes Regulations. This has resulted in significant activity being commissioned through PMS Plus:

- 2500 new referrals in a range of specialties are managed in-house per annum. This accounts for more than 90 per cent of the partnership's total elective referrals in these areas.
- Two suitably accredited GPs carry out 340 minor surgical procedures each year. These procedures would all fall outside the criteria of GMS/PMS minor surgery and would otherwise have required referral to a surgeon.
- More than 2500 plain film X-rays and 700 non-invasive ultrasounds are carried out each year.
- 200 gastroscopies are also performed in the attached day surgery unit, the service being co-ordinated with that of the local trusts to make sure that the two-week cancer guidelines are adhered to.

The majority of these services are provided from the unit attached to one of the practice sites, though the ultrasonographer and the dietician, for example, hold clinics at both sites.

The benefits of PMS Plus

The PMS Plus pilot has delivered a number of benefits for patients, including:

- Reduced attendance at the A&E department for urgent X-rays through provision of in-house services (in 2000/01, roughly 140 patients received this service).
- A reduced follow-up ratio for specialist outpatients. The pilot now manages a 'new to follow-up' ratio of 1:2, whereas under fundholding this ratio was 1:4 (although the latter figure includes all specialties).
- A maximum wait for gastroscopy of four weeks (although approximately 90 per cent are carried out within two weeks).
- Assessment and pre-referral 'work-up' of potential referrals in relation to ENT, urology, diabetes and paediatrics by designated 'sub-specialist' GPs prior to onward transmission to a hospital consultant. Where appropriate, cases are managed in-house.

As well as providing better patient care, the pilot has delivered significant cost savings. The reduction in specialist follow-up care has saved significant resources (in 2001/02 every outpatient appointment costs £56.00). Rapid diagnostic advice in relation to upper gastrointestinal complaints has led to more cost-effective prescribing. The partnership prescribes proton pump inhibitors at a rate significantly below the national average. Financial surpluses made during total purchasing and the PMS pilot have been ploughed back into practice-based patient services. Since 1995, the number of GPs working within the partnership has risen from 9.4 WTE to 13 WTE. Similarly, there has been a significant rise in the number of nurses employed, particularly in relation to the care of diabetics and the provision of clinics for rheumatology and respiratory and cardiovascular disease. In addition, it has also been possible to achieve a reasonable improvement in the profitability of the business to the benefit of the partners.

Managing a multi-practice organisation

ICP has become large and increasingly complex. A new management structure was established (see Figure 6.2).

The strategic management of the pilot is co-ordinated by the partnership executive, which consists of two partners and the general manager. Each partner also takes responsibility for a particular area of interest (finance, IT, human resources, etc.) and feeds proposals for developments into the executive. All policy decisions go to the full partnership board, which operates in a 'cabinet' structure. In this way, the different interests and abilities of the partners are harnessed to the benefit of all and the workload is reasonably distributed.

Figure 6.2 Management of the PMS pilot

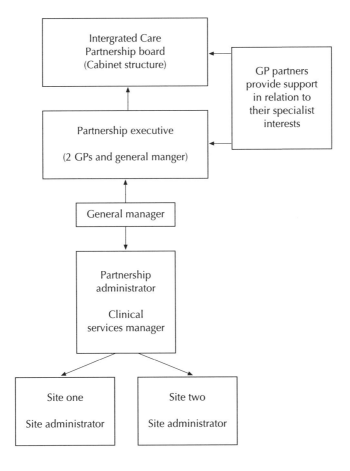

The general manager's role is predominantly financial and strategic, but includes the line management of a clinical services manager (who is responsible for the operational side of the PMS Plus services) and the partnership administrator (who provides the human resources function as well as being responsible, with the help of two site administrators, for the PMS services). While the management of a large multi-site organisation is inevitably more complicated than that of the traditional 'stand alone' general practice, it does provide new opportunities to strengthen the management function. By combining the practice management resources, economies of scale have been achieved – the whole is greater than the sum of the parts.

Naturally, with such a merger and expansion, the partnership obtained good legal advice over its PMS contracts, in particular ensuring that any workload additional to that of GMS/PMS was reimbursed. The practice has also introduced a new partnership agreement, written with legal advice.

Relationships with the health authority and PCG

Before the merger, the respective practices had always been at the forefront of primary care provision in East Surrey and had been ably and willingly supported by the health authority through fundholding and total purchasing. Over the years, a good two-way relationship had developed – the practices, being in the first wave of most initiatives, often had the benefit of being involved with setting any new ground rules, and the health authority had a willing test-bed for new ideas.

The introduction of the PCG complicated matters. Although the PCG is supportive of the ICP, the process of evolution is often frustrated by increased bureaucracy and the need for conformity across the group. The PCG, however, remains very much dominated by the health authority, which is itself under constant regional office pressure to fulfil the multitude of political initiatives and priorities. Fortunately, improving patient care – in particular developing better local access, GP specialisation, increasing nursing activity, booked surgery admissions and reduced waiting lists – are all government priorities outlined in the NHS Plan. The ICP has been achieving all of these since 1998, so should continue to build on this success. The relationship with the PCG will almost certainly change further once it achieves PCT status, at which point we may have to move our contract from the health authority.

A significant issue has been that of conflict of interest. The ICP has, in essence, purchased services from among its own members, and the day surgery unit is privately owned by the GPs. The pilot has been careful to ensure that all contracts have been formally between the partnership and the health authority, and all interests have been declared.

In 1998/9, the pilot applied successfully to the Secretary of State to extend its PMS pilot to more specialties. In most cases, patients treated under the PMS Plus contract were offered a booked admission date for surgery at the outpatient assessment, with waits usually of less than three months. Where these contracts remain with acute trusts, under the large block contracts agreed with the PCG and health authorities this is not the case. In addition, full funding has continued to pass to trusts, even though activity has fallen significantly and waiting lists have risen. Sadly, two years after their approval, these contract extensions are still held up by the health authority, PCG and trusts due to difficulties in shifting the financial resources. It is hoped these contracts will soon be taken over by the partnership under PMS Plus, where we will not get contract income if we fail to perform. This will provide greater incentives for efficiency and more scope to use our resources creatively and effectively to maximise patient care.

The future

Local practices are now considering the formation of a non-profit-making limited company that includes the ICP in order to extend the benefits of PMS to more patients: outpatient waiting times of eight weeks or less; gastroscopy waiting times of two weeks for urgent and a maximum of three to four weeks for routine; and three to four month maximum waiting times for booked admissions for day surgery. Our experience to date suggests that the population covered by the ICP is too small to plan and deliver all services that might usefully be made more local. We expect the ideal population for this to be in the region of 70,000 to 80,000. We are exploring the possibility of the new, larger network of practices carrying out a wide range of PMS Plus provision on a locality-wide basis.

In the immediate future, we hope to expand our PMS Plus services (together with our neighbouring practices) to include intermediate inpatient and home care. This might cover as much as 40 to 50 per cent of acute hospital inpatient care that is currently purchased. We would also like to develop GP and nurse minor injuries and immediately necessary care services, and make them available until 11 p.m. This would incorporate walk-in services, leading to improved access for patients to non-urgent care. These, of course, require resourcing and will need contracts to support infrastructure, management and additional medical and nursing inputs.

Lessons from the first wave

At present, cost pressures on the acute services are providing the greatest obstacle to developing services. Unfortunately, they are currently unable to cope. As a consequence, we believe that local control of service delivery is essential. While PCTs are to be generally welcomed, these new organisations may prove too large to exercise the degree of control over clinical activity that has been achieved by the PMS pilot.

We certainly believe we have delivered most of the NHS Plan objectives well ahead of the Plan being written. While much of our infrastructure was developed during the fundholding and total purchasing era, it is PMS (and in particular PMS Plus) that has allowed us to simplify arrangements for the direct provision of an extended range of services. This has not only allowed us to retain existing patient services, but also to build on them and now expand them gradually to patients of the other practices in the locality.

Chapter 7

Commissioning PMS pilots – the health authority view

Rigo Pizarro-Duhart

KEY POINTS

Lambeth, Southwark and Lewisham Health Authority has seen a dramatic expansion of PMS coverage. Much has been learnt in the process of developing over 100 new practice-based contracts. Appropriate performance management presents a major challenge.

Introduction

Lambeth, Southwark and Lewisham (LSL) Health Authority, in south-east London, contains one of the largest PMS pilot programmes in the country. PMS pilots have become one of the main mechanisms for the delivery of primary care services locally and provide the impetus for development and change within general practice.

The reasons for such a large-scale movement from the national GMS arrangements to a PMS contract are complex. The explanation must partly be found in the local history of primary care development in the area, as well as in the concerns and expectations of GPs following the publication of the *New NHS* White Paper and the emergence of PCGs and PCTs. Certainly, local strategic vision and the proactive approach taken by the health authority and PCGs also played a role. The end result is a new landscape in which a majority of practices are PMS pilots operating under a local contract and subject to performance management. This may have far-reaching implications for the development and the provision of primary care in south-east London as PCGs move towards PCT status.

The scope of the programme

Only four first wave proposals went forward for approval by the Secretary of State. Moreover, these PMS proposals could not be said to be typical of general practice as a whole. For example, two of them were led by local community trusts and another by Guys' and St Thomas's NHS Hosptial Trust. The only practice-based proposal involved a group of GPs who were already salaried to the local medical school.

In the second wave, 27 proposals involving 34 practices were approved by the Secretary of State. These new pilots raised the proportion of local GPs working under PMS contracts within the health authority to 26 per cent, and the share of the population registered with a PMS practice to nearly 30 per cent (see Table 7.1). The overwhelming majority of pilots were practice-based pilots, with only one proposal led by the local community trust.

While the interest generated by the second wave took everybody by surprise, the third wave has gone a step further – 32 pilots incorporating 45 practices went live in April 2001, with another 18 pilots ready to commence in October 2001. If all of these pilots go live, then two-thirds of all GPs in LSL and more than 72 per cent of the registered population will be within the scheme. Within three years, PMS has become the predominant mode of primary care contracting.

Perhaps one of the main achievements of the programme has been the successful bid for new salaried GPs and nurse practitioners (see Table 7.2). Applications for additional resources were accepted because the health authority is deemed to be 'under-doctored' (with a high patient to doctor ratio) when compared to the national average, and because the quality of many of the proposals was high. Proposals highlighted specific local needs that are not easily recognised or met using GMS contracting. In all, the health authority has received £4.06m (2001/02 prices) recurring resources for additional primary care clinical staff – a significant boost to local services.

A large majority of the pilots have practice-based contracts, and the GPs leaving GMS will remain independent contractors. All pilots have elected to become 'NHS bodies' and will therefore use NHS contracts (or

Table 7.1 PMS pilots in Lambeth, Southwark and Lewisham Health Authority

	First Wave		Second Wave		Third Wave (a)		Third Wave (b)		Total	
	No.	%	No.	%	No.	%	No.	%	No.	%
PMS pilots	4	N/A	27	N/A	32	N/A	18	N/A	81	N/A
Practices in PMS pilots	4	2.3	34	21.0	45	28.0	19	11.8	102	63.1
GPs (WTE)	15	3.3	111	22.8	125	27.9	56	12.5	307	66.5
Population	12,881	1.6	235,252	27.5	265,127	31.1	103,231	12.1	616,491	72.3

WTE = whole time equivalent

Table 7.2 Additional medical and nursing workforce through PMS pilots

	First wave	Second wave	Third wave (a)	Third wave (b)	Total
New WTE salaried GPs	5	18	24	10	57
New WTE nurse practitioners	1	4	13	4	22

WTE= whole time equivalent

Table 7.3 Objectives of PMS pilots

Objectives	First wave	Second wave	Third wave
Sexual health	–	10	17
Mental health	1	9	21
Drugs and alcohol	–	9	11
Refugees and ethnic minorities	1	9	14
Elderly services	–	6	18
Children and young people	–	5	13
Homeless people	–	4	4
Deprived communities	4	15	28
Travellers	–	1	0

Note: The table shows the total number of objectives identified. Pilots have selected more than one objective.

'service agreements') to determine their relationship with the NHS. However, while general practice has remained largely unchanged in terms of the employment status of GPs, PMS has introduced a rich variety of organisational arrangements and service models. In particular, practices are now working collaboratively with each other and with other agencies. Some examples are set out in Box 7.1.

The local context

Arguably, there has been a whole range of motives behind this unprecedented level of GP interest in the PMS programme. This level of motivation is at least partly the product of the recent history of primary care development in the area. The PMS programme followed in the footsteps of a large London Initiative Zone (LIZ) programme – a developmental initiative instigated by the Tomlinson Inquiry into London's health care. This injected significant resources into the primary care infrastructure between 1993 and 1999. The health authority had

---

BOX 7.1 ORGANISATIONAL AND SERVICE DELIVERY INNOVATIONS

- One pilot is 'nurse-led', managed by the community trust.
- Eight pilots, involving 28 practices, have formed multi-practice organisations. This has particularly involved single-handed practices that are now grouping together to provide services.
- Seven single-handed or small practices in South Lewisham are sharing organisational resources and services, such as practice managers and nurses, and provide specialist services to each others' patients (e.g. family planning and minor surgery).
- Two single-handed practices in Lambeth are supported by a large group practice within the locality to form a single primary care organisation.
- One PMS pilot serves as the focus for a community-wide children and nutrition project.
- One PMS pilot works with local schools to provide family planning and counselling services to school children who may not be registered patients.
- One PMS pilot has developed a new participatory structure for its staff and developed a system of incentives and staff appraisals around major PMS objectives.
- A group of PMS pilots pool resources together with the community trust to provide a comprehensive service to refugees and asylum seekers.
- One pilot serves as the base for an integrated health and social care team for the elderly for the whole PCG.
- One pilot proposes to provide services for Vietnamese refugees in a deprived area.

---

already developed local development schemes and a range of agreed service and quality indicators for use in allocating resources (including a 'banding system' that differentiated between levels of practice performance). A large number of second wave PMS applicants had achieved the higher banding levels and were therefore confident in signing up to local contracts.

It is also clear that the notion of replacing the GMS contract (known as the 'terms of service' and the 'Red Book') by a block contract was attractive to GPs, who felt overwhelmed by bureaucracy or felt constrained by the inflexibility of national payment arrangements. The levels of deprivation and the specific needs of inner city populations (including the high proportion of refugees and homeless people) had long been inadequately resourced under GMS.

However, motives were rather more complex than this. At the time the second wave of PMS pilots was announced, PCGs were forming and chief executives had only just been appointed. PMS were seen by many GPs as a way to influence the terms of their relationship with these new bodies during a period of change and uncertainty.

PCGs and strategic fit

PCGs raised some initial concerns about the implications of PMS on their ability to manage primary care as well as on their unified budgets (given the controlling role of the health authority and the fact that PMS contracts were partly funded from local contracts). There was widespread anxiety about loss of control and practices 'opting out' from their PCGs, though this perception has (so far at least) proved unfounded.

PMS also developed within a context of very limited resource growth, especially for primary care. This made it difficult for PCGs to meet PMS proposals that required resources for additional practice staffing or some of the most innovative PMS Plus proposals that required additional Hospital and Community Health Services (HCHS) funding (the latter could only be shifted from the community services or secondary sector).

As a result, it became crucially important that colleagues in the PCGs and within the health authority understood the goals, nature and process of the PMS programme. The question was whether PMS pilots offered a strategic opportunity or, rather, a hindrance to other developments. The health authority engaged in an intensive strategic debate, both internally and with PCGs, on how PMS fitted with the plans to modernise the NHS. The outcome of this debate was that the PMS programme would be encouraged both to support the development of PCGs and to test out new organisational arrangements as the transition to PCT status took place.

The process

The sheer scale of the programme confronted the health authority and colleagues in the PCGs with a number of difficult logistical problems. This had serious management implications, not least how the PMS contracts could be negotiated with so many individual pilots at once.

Conversely, how would it be possible to agree a contract acceptable to all without losing sight of the individual aspirations and creativity that should underpin the concept of a local contract?

The answer to both questions had to be a pragmatic one. The approach adopted in LSL involved dividing up the contract into three levels:

- national or core requirements
- local (PCG-level) strategic requirements
- pilot-specific objectives.

Core elements were negotiated collectively across the health authority, whereas PCGs were empowered to agree locality-level and practice-specific issues. Financial issues would be handled on a one-to-one basis by the health authority (for non-cash-limited baselines) and by the PCGs (for discretionary items such as practice staffing).

At this point, it must be said that the successes of this approach depended largely on the process that was followed. The perception was that all the stakeholders were embarking on a journey into the unknown and therefore it was imperative to create an environment of participation and consultation rather than confrontation. The health authority and the PCGs spent a great deal of time and effort involving key GPs and decision-makers in the planning process. Critically, at each phase in the development of the programme (producing proposals, writing business plans, agreeing a contract), GPs and other members of the primary care team were invited to attend workshops and conferences that facilitated the dialogue and established direct lines of communication. As a result, most GPs felt consulted on the major issues and the quality of the information improved. This avoided misunderstandings and prevented the ill-informed gossip that tends to replace reality in some circumstances.

Above all, this cycle of seminars and workshops allowed GPs and their staff to compare notes and to develop their own leadership structure, which became known as the Contract Development Working Group for the second wave of pilots. This was an *ad hoc* group of GPs, nurses and practice managers that emerged to represent the wider group of pilots.

Later, this group was joined by advisors from the BMA. While the LMC played a limited role at this stage, the working group kept them informed of developments.

The working group negotiated the contract detail with the health authority. It was agreed that, having done the preliminary work, the contract would be handed over to the health authority solicitors and solicitors acting independently for the working group to finalise. The involvement of legal advisors was controversial: the NHS Executive discouraged this as an unnecessary and expensive process to agree what was, after all, an NHS contract and not a legally binding document. However, the legal input proved to be very helpful in reassuring GPs, and indeed the health authority, that the new contractual and accountability framework was fair and safe. Notwithstanding the involvement of lawyers, the working group increasingly moved away from a posture of 'negotiation' to one of collaboration and common ownership of the contract. This was undoubtedly one of the most important reasons for the success of the programme.

A very similar approach was adopted for the third wave, notwithstanding the introduction of the national contractual framework for PMS. A new contract development steering group was set up with the active participation of the LMC and PCGs. This project structure has helped maintain the atmosphere of collaboration and trust. Above all, many of the issues that had seemed complex or politically difficult in the previous round were now settled. Stakeholders felt confident enough to enable the LMC and the health authority to settle the detail of the new contract. The local contract proved sufficiently robust to cope with the demands of the increasingly prescriptive Department of Health. In particular, the new PMS national contractual framework, which incorporates the requirements, targets and standards of the NHS Plan, is now absorbed into the core contractual requirements, while still leaving space for local discretion and creativity.

The structure of the contract

From the point of view of the GPs, there were a number of important issues to consider, including: the terms and conditions for providing PMS services; the statutory and clinical responsibilities of the contracting parties; the financial framework; and performance management.

Terms and conditions

Unsurprisingly, many GPs chose to focus on the implications of moving from one legal and regulatory framework into another. This meant that the working group spent a great deal of time seeking or producing clarification on so-called 'core issues' dealing with definitions, legal obligations, conditions for the termination of contracts, action in case of default, arbitration, legal liabilities, etc. It can be argued that a lot of this was already well established in the various Department of Health directions and regulations. However, in order to address anxieties and place these regulations in a clearer context, a large portion of the contract turned into a commentary on these issues.

Responsibilities of parties to the contract

GPs were keen to clarify their professional responsibilities and relationships in the new environment. This pertained mainly to the establishment of clear definitions of who the patients were and how they would be registered, the clinical responsibilities of salaried doctors, and the clinical liabilities of the rest of the team. One interesting point (that has yet to be resolved) is the management of disciplinary matters and whether this is an issue of individual GP responsibility or the responsibility of the pilot as a whole as part of its contractual obligations.

The financial framework

The financial framework is a key foundation of the contract. Perhaps surprisingly, once the process for agreeing baselines and contract prices had been established, financial issues were less controversial than had originally been expected. This is not to say, however, that there was not a great deal of 'haggling' going on on an individual basis over specific items. There was also widespread disappointment about the lack of additional resources available to fund some of the most interesting service developments previously described. Unsurprisingly, while the approval of proposals by the Secretary of State raised expectations locally, disappointment was only partly offset by the success of the programme in securing growth for additional salaried GPs.

The main collective preoccupation involved issues of risk management. For example, GPs tended to focus on issues such as the impact of sudden, new cost pressures or unexpected reductions of activity (e.g. a fall in list size). Would these result in a variation of contract and/or a reduction in practice profitability? This required confidence in the contracting process and a degree of mutual trust that could be built only over a long period of time.

One area of contention between health authority and pilots (that ultimately could not be resolved) was in relation to the critical issue of financial accountability and individual GP income. The health authority originally offered a contract that established a 'floor' and a 'ceiling' on GP income. GP personal income was not expected to rise or fall more than 10 per cent compared to its historic GMS position. The objective was to ensure transparency and financial control over budget surpluses in exchange for financial security (i.e. pilots would be protected from significant income loss). While the idea attracted some interest, most GPs saw this as threatening their independent contractor status and resisted the idea. In the end, the health authority settled for a system whereby only discretionary items and targeted resources (e.g. allocated growth for GP salaries) would be scrutinised routinely and underspends be clawed back. However, GPs also undertook to abide internally by a set of financial control systems developed by the health authority and would be open to financial audit.

Performance management

Performance management of the contract also proved controversial. The concept as originally presented constituted a cultural shock to many practitioners. The health authority was anxious to develop a firm and comprehensive accountability framework, supported by the collection of performance-related data. However, this health authority objective was in tension with other key purposes of PMS pilots – to be rid of the Red Book and a reduction in bureaucracy. There was widespread concern about the practicality of the proposed accountability framework and whether both parties would have sufficient resources to maintain the process. In the end, a pragmatic solution was found: it was agreed that core performance management would be focused on a number of objectives and targets set by the pilot as part of its business plan. These would reflect the individual proposals as well as wider local (PCG) requirements. Where possible, the performance indicators would be qualitative and outcome based. In addition, PMS pilots would be scrutinised for their contribution to the objectives of local primary care investment plans (PCIPs) and health improvement plans (HImPs). Finally, pilots would be assessed against national standards and targets contained within a minimum data set applied to all pilots.

The issue of capacity has been significant in relation to performance management. The health authority has not had sufficient capacity to manage ongoing relationships with so many pilots (although this is not our role in any case). However, PCGs, to which performance management responsibilities have been delegated, have also struggled. PMS is one of many competing objectives. The developmental approach that should underpin the commissioner–provider relationship requires more managerial resources than have so far been available. Performance management is becoming more sophisticated, but to date we have been unable to deliver all that is necessary.

Developmental support for pilots

The health authority has developed a number of standard tools and developmental interventions to support prospective pilots and ensure they are well prepared to go live.

Organisational development checklist

An organisational development (OD) 'checklist' was designed with three main purposes:

- to help identify gaps in the development of the pilots (e.g. lack of adequate information systems)
- to provide a tool for the assessment of potential risks (e.g. employment law, inadequate premises, health and safety problems, clinical risks, etc.)
- to help set basic organisational standards designed to enhance quality (e.g. every pilot must have staff and clinical meetings, practice managers must hold a qualification, etc.).

Each practice carried out a self-assessment and shared the results with the health authority and PCG, both of which were able to offer developmental support.

Business plan

The business plan emerged as the core document designed to test out and give shape to initial proposals, develop more specific, measurable and achievable objectives, and provide a local basis for performance management. Each business plan had to be agreed between the pilot and its PCG, offering the possibility for more detailed negotiations to fine-tune proposals around local (PCG/PCIP) priorities, often linked to the application of discretionary (cash-limited) resources controlled by the PCG. The business plan also encouraged pilots to think through how their sometimes very ambitious plans might be phased over the lifetime of the pilot. The developmental process did not cease once the pilot went live.

Financial systems assessment

The OD checklist was complemented by a financial systems assessment tool dealing with financial controls, budgeting and financial information systems. On these bases, the health authority developed some guidelines for financial reporting and control that were annexed to the contract. These guidelines were produced with the support of the health authority's internal auditors, and established basic principles for financial management at practice level, focusing on the task of supervising a cash-limited block contract. The proposed system incorporated notions of budget holding, reconciliation and reporting. It was facilitated by the application of standard software, and the health authority offered a simple off-the-shelf package free to those who were not well acquainted with these methods.

Conclusion

The experience of the PMS programme in LSL is very rich. It has provoked important cultural and organisational change and has opened the way for a more flexible, dynamic and collaborative environment in which both professionals and services can develop to the benefit of patients.

But there are a number of caveats. The process has lacked investment in service development, and the resources for organisational development are also limited. In addition, many of the arrangements for performance management and evaluation remain fragile at best, with the constant risk of losing track of progress. A key issue has been that of insufficient managerial resources at commissioner level, as well as a lack of protected practitioners' time to focus on project management and delivery. As a result, many of the benefits cannot yet be realised, and where they have it has proved difficult to extract the necessary learning or to share these experiences in a systematic way.

Nevertheless, both GPs and managers have begun to recognise PMS as a flexible developmental tool of great potential. In addition, it may represent a potential solution to the dilemma faced since the inception of PCGs and inherent in the accountability structure of PCTs – how to facilitate the integration of independent contractors such as GPs within a local structure of public accountability. The answer seems obvious: provide GPs with local contracts held by the PCTs.

There are also other crucial questions that remain unanswered. For example, the issue of the future affordability of PMS as primary care becomes increasingly funded through local cash-limited budgets. Additional growth for PMS comes from a single pot that is allocated at national level. It can be argued that PMS has encouraged some redistribution of resources to inner city areas such as Lambeth, Southwark and Lewisham, but this must have consequences for other areas. In addition, with the introduction of a new resource allocation for primary care resources imminent, can we be sure that these resource streams will continue to flow?

There is a further question about the implications of such a large PMS programme for the remaining GMS practices. Already some perceive a degree of inequity as PMS practices secure large amounts of funding for employing salaried GPs. These funding streams are simply not available upfront to GMS practices. Certainly, PMS are serving as a spur to review the working of the GP national contract and bring these two contracts more into line as suggested by the NHS Plan.

There are many lessons to learn from these pilots and it may even be argued that the primary care in this part of south London is now poised to make the qualitative leap to a new form of service delivery. As yet this is an aspiration rather than reality. The vision of flexible and well-integrated primary care services operating within the context of local public health and organisational strategies remains to be achieved.

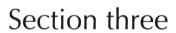

Section three

Chapter 8

Conclusion

Personal medical services – modernising primary care?

Richard Lewis and Stephen Gillam

The first wave of PMS pilots have completed their first three years. The vast majority of them are still operating – once achieving 'live' status few pilots have reverted to GMS or ceased trading altogether. This, in itself, is some sort of achievement.

The first wave of pilots has provided a rich source of learning about PMS, and evaluations have begun to report their findings. Yet, inevitably, it still feels rather early to judge the impact of PMS pilots on primary care. Furthermore, learning from first wave pilots may not be transferable to later waves. This sits uneasily with the Government's early decision to encourage a wide take-up of the scheme. The vast majority of pilots have entered the scheme in the third wave and under very different conditions.

A clear message from the King's Fund case studies is that, in many respects, PMS pilots have not introduced radical changes to existing practice. Many of those developments that have occurred are difficult to attribute directly to PMS (what we refer to below as a 'PMS effect'). For existing GMS practitioners, life in a PMS pilot may not seem all that different. Is that a failure of PMS? Not if PMS provides a vehicle for gradual yet sustained development.

What other conclusions can one reach about the success, or otherwise, of PMS pilots? The expectations for the scheme were high but PMS pilots alone will not 'modernise' primary care. However, we believe that there are four dimensions of primary care where PMS pilots are particularly suited to delivering the Government's modernisation objectives:

- local contracting
- service quality
- tackling inequalities
- development of new clinical roles and organisational structures.

We pose questions below in relation to each of these and consider the evidence.

Have local contracts led to more responsive primary care?

The replacement of the national GP contract with a series of locally negotiated service agreements has been a key feature of the PMS movement. The limitations of the Red Book are well known. By focusing on the 'average', it fails to recognise the very different needs of different populations. In particular, it has a perverse ability (in certain circumstances) to financially reward poor-quality care. In theory, PMS pilots provide the perfect antidote. Initially, pilots were encouraged to write their contracts from scratch, constrained only by their imagination. Significant national growth money was made available to enable new, highly targeted services to be commissioned.

And yet early evaluations of the local contracting process showed a disappointing take-up of these new flexibilities.[1,2] Pilot service agreements included few outcome-oriented measures. Indeed, the most common indicators used looked remarkably like those so familiar to GMS doctors. Nor were the contracts seen as dynamic tools, flexibly focusing pilot activities year-on-year. In the King's Fund case studies, only one pilot reviewed its contract structure during the three years of the pilot and there is no reason to believe this to be untypical. Moreover, nationally the contract monitoring process is variable and felt by some to be ineffective.[3]

It is tempting to conclude that local contracting itself has had little impact on the nature of the service provided. Why is this? First wave pilots were largely driven by the providers themselves. As we previously reported, commissioners were reactive rather than proactive agents, and had other objectives to achieve.[4] As Clare Jenkins describes, some health authorities viewed their pilots as 'piranhas' and saw risks rather than opportunities. These are unlikely to be the conditions under which serious contract negotiations will be undertaken. The approach adopted in south-east London, described by Rigo Pizarro-Duhart, has been unusual: the commissioning health authority could not remain passive given the rapid penetration of PMS. However, even with this motivation, capacity issues have proved significant. Holding local pilots to account using individually tailored contracts requires more resources than are usually available at commissioner level.

The existence of a 'return ticket' to GMS for most GP PMS providers is also likely to impede the extent to which commissioners might use a contract as a means to exact compliance. As to how long this ticket will be valid is another question. With permanence arrangements soon to be announced, the decision to switch into PMS may become irrevocable. Finally, there is the issue of the prevailing culture. This has hardly been supportive of the notion of contracting. PMS pilots were introduced at exactly the time that the Government had pronounced the 'death of the NHS internal market'. Our case studies suggest that pilots and their commissioners preferred a more developmental relationship to that which is implied by agent–principal theory. In situations of 'high trust', contracts may be redundant.[5]

However, it is in the area of contracting that the Government has proved itself most willing to act. By the third wave of pilots a new contractual structure was introduced. A 'national contractual framework' is now mandatory for all aspiring pilots. This framework set down key indicators that all pilots have to achieve. These reflect government priorities and are demanding. For example, all pilots have to meet higher GMS targets for cervical cancer screening and childhood immunisation, and provide access to a clinician within 24 hours of request and to a GP within 48 hours. The national contractual framework also specifies that pilots must meet all the primary care requirements of the national service frameworks (NSFs) – something of a blank cheque, given that NSFs are continuing to be developed.

Notwithstanding the core requirements laid down by the Department of Health, pilots are mandated to develop local pilot-specific contract objectives. In principle, this balance between central direction and local discretion appears a sensible strategy. The result, however, is a PMS scheme that looks very different in its adolescence than it did in its infancy.

Of course, there is also a highly political dimension to this fundamental change to the primary care contract. The introduction of local contracts has significant implications for government–profession relations. Surprisingly, it has taken three years for the BMA to challenge overtly the loss of negotiating rights in relation to PMS pilots. Now, this issue is at the centre of the festering dispute between organised medical interests and the Department of Health. The NHS Plan has made clear that the GMS contract is to be brought in line with PMS, and contractual convergence appears imminent.

Have PMS pilots improved quality of care?

A central concern driving the earliest consultations leading up to the 1997 NHS (Primary Care) Act was the need to find ways of tailoring local contracts to local needs. The first guidance stressed the importance of ensuring care of high clinical quality. The following dimensions of quality were singled out: effectiveness, efficiency, accessibility and responsiveness.

A rigorous assessment of the impact of these pilots requires a controlled trial matching PMS and non-PMS sites, and such a study has been undertaken as part of the national evaluation. To what extent do our more-limited case studies accord with the findings of others? And what do they tell us about quality of care under PMS?

The definition and measurement of quality in primary care is notoriously problematic. The best-validated measures focus on the processes of chronic disease management. These may be difficult to link to changes in health outcomes that usually require longer-term monitoring. High on patients' lists of priorities are communications skills and the opportunity to form trusting relationships with their doctor or nurse. These aspects of quality are not easily assessed nor specified in contracts. We employed the measures used by the national evaluation team, thereby allowing cross comparisons.

The interim report from the national evaluation compares 23 first wave PMS practices in 19 pilots with a similar sample of matched non-PMS practices. They examined the same range of quality indicators and concluded, at that stage, that there was little detectable difference in quality of provision. Interestingly, in some key respects PMS pilots began with a lower-quality baseline than the GMS controls. This runs counter to the often-held view that early adopters tend to be the best, seeking to improve further.[6]

Our work similarly finds little strong or consistent evidence of a 'PMS effect' on quality. This is unsurprising, given the measurement difficulties referred to and short timescales, but is nonetheless disappointing. Few interviewees gave testimony to dramatic improvements. Both of the established sites involved practices where standards were, for the most part, already high.

What can one conclude from all of this? First, PMS has not revolutionised quality of practice; it would be unrealistic to hope that it would. Instead, quality improvements in existing practices are likely to be more incremental. There was, for example, some evidence in Hillingdon that the formation of a new partnership involving salaried practice in formerly single-handed practices helped raise standards of organisation and clinical care. With new, trust-led pilots, the 'PMS effect' was more obvious – without the pilot there would be no service. In our two 'new practice' case studies, objective measurement of quality was problematic. However, focus groups confirmed positive differences to the traditional experience of general practice. Tim Crossley, in his description of the Wolverhampton PMS scheme, strongly affirms the benefits of a larger-scale initiative tackling quality in previously isolated practices. This represents a major advance.

The nurse-led sites serving new lists are the most intriguing. As far as we could tell, in the face of periodic staffing discontinuities, the quality of technical care was maintained in the Edith Cavell Practice. However, by comparison with the national PMS sample, some patients clearly experienced difficulties gaining timely access to their carer of choice. Catharine Baraniak and Lance Gardner, on the other hand, claim personal care and continuity as a particular strength of their pilots (although more evidence is required to substantiate these claims). Problems stemming from impaired continuity of care would surely arise on any site experiencing rapid staff turnover and upheaval.

The broader experience of the national and King's Fund evaluations does suggest that, while salaried posts are appealing for the post holder, many doctors employed on three-year contracts will move on. For those patients whose expectation is of a long-term relationship, this is bound to be unsatisfactory.

The final dimension – that of efficiency – is still harder to call. The first wave PMS pilots received more generous financial allocations than their successors. The national evaluation found each pilot received, on average, an additional £62,000 compared to their previous, non-pilot year. No comparative data are as yet available, so it is difficult to put this gain into context.[7]

The trust-led sites serving smaller, needier lists bear particularly high costs per capita. These were seen as inefficient in the eyes of other doctors. PCTs face difficult decisions over future funding for such projects. They should keep in mind that, ethical considerations apart, the 'hidden' costs of inappropriate secondary care, A&E usage and poor primary care may still outweigh extra investment in primary care. Certainly, the experience of both the St Hilary Brow Practice in the Wirral and the Epsom Integrated Care Partnership suggests that a significant proportion of hospital work can be relocated to primary care. James Kingsland, together with his health authority, demonstrated that a substantial investment in primary care was more than repaid through savings at the hospital door. In this case, PMS has delivered efficiency, primary care development and patient satisfaction – a heady mix indeed.

In essence, the balance of costs and benefits involves trade-offs. In the right hands, in the right organisational circumstances and under sensitive management, we have evidence that PMS *can* improve quality of care.

Have PMS pilots reduced inequalities in access to primary care?

Concerns over how better primary care could be delivered to populations that have historically been poorly served provided a *raison d'être* to differing extents at all four sites we investigated. The extent to which GPs are centrally concerned about the needs of their practice population 'beyond the surgery door' is debatable. This touches on a central ethical challenge for today's general practitioner. While traditionally individualistic in their focus – on the needs of the patient consulting – they are being required to adopt more utilitarian approaches to decision-making in the interests of a broader practice or even PCT population. The nurse-led sites were set up to serve particularly needy populations. While only a small minority had not previously been registered, it seems likely that patients from black and minority ethnic groups, including refugees and asylum seekers and homeless people, have received more effective care from their PMS practices. One reason for this is that the community trusts brought additional resources to the table, for example access to interpreting services and other relevant voluntary organisations. The siting of practices alongside other providers was of benefit. As discussed above, the extent to which this is cost-efficient is untested.

However, attempts in existing practices to increase provision for people with mental health problems or older people were less successful (at least within the timeframe of our evaluation). Where the PMS pilot involved established work patterns, the final product was indistinguishable from traditional GMS – notwithstanding the rhetoric of the original proposals.

At the very least, first wave pilots tend to be located in more deprived areas. This suggests that PMS has been used to address issues of health inequality. Rigo Pizarro-Duhart testifies to a wide range of projects targeting vulnerable populations. This is substantiated by the national evaluation, together with evidence of a 'community development' approach to pilot implementation.[8,9] Lance Gardner described the approach adopted by the Daruzzaman Care Centre in Salford. Here, members of the local community form a board of trustees that oversee his PMS pilot.

Yet some interesting ethical issues are raised. In our case studies and in the evaluation of nurse-led pilots, anecdotal evidence suggests that 'mainstream' general practices began to direct certain patient groups (such as refugees) towards PMS practices. In some respects this is to be expected and welcomed. After all, these pilots have been deliberately established to serve vulnerable populations. They have an infrastructure that is skilled, willing and able to meet the particular needs. However, it raises significant issues of choice. Should not refugees or homeless people also have a choice of practice? Are we creating 'ghetto primary care' and letting other practices 'off the hook'?

Observers are likely to have been struck by the allocation to PMS pilots of significant growth monies. These have not been available (at least not in the same way and with the same flexibility) to GMS practices. New salaried GPs (and now nurse practitioners) have come into post in significant numbers. However, they can been seen as largely 'free goods' to the practices that receive them. This may not be perceived as fair by GMS and PMS practices alike. Indeed, the methodology for allocating these growth funds has been unclear. PMS is limited to volunteers; the extent to which PMS can address existing resource inequities must always be hit-and-miss. We have commented elsewhere on the perverse outcomes that the co-existence of PMS and GMS might deliver.[10] The single resource allocation framework, announced in the NHS Plan, is urgently needed.

Has PMS led to the development of new roles and organisational forms?

It is in this dimension that PMS pilots have clearly been seen to deliver. The national and other evaluations have suggested that nursing roles in particular have been developed within pilots.[11,12] An admittedly extreme example of this is provided by the nine first wave 'nurse-led' pilots. Here, nurses have handled much 'first contact' work and provided clinical and managerial leadership. In his evaluation of the nine first wave pilots, Richard Lewis suggests that they have been remarkably successful in inverting the traditional hierarchy between doctors and nurses. In these pilots, nurses now routinely refer patients directly to hospital consultants or for diagnostic tests. The term 'nurse-led', however, may confuse as much as it illuminates. 'Nurse leads' have adopted this label simply to distinguish themselves from 'traditional' general practice. Their goal is a primary care team without hierarchy, in which all professionals may use their skills to the full. Patients, it seems, are less concerned whether a service is provided by a nurse or a doctor, so long as it provides social support and continuity of care.[13]

Notwithstanding their successes, nurse-led pilots faced difficulties and resistance, particularly from local medical colleagues. Nurse-led primary care is by no means an easy option, as evidenced by the testimony of Catherine Baraniak and Lance Gardner.

In our case studies, nurses have been broadly positive about their opportunities within PMS. However, there has been less evidence of concrete examples of distinct changes to the professional roles of team members. The experience of the Edith Cavell pilot has demonstrated that such radical changes to practice are not easily achieved and may be bruising for those concerned.

New organisational forms have abounded. PMS appears to have stimulated growth in the size of the practice unit; numerous examples of this have been presented in this book. The South West London Primary Care Organisation and the Integrated Care Partnership in Epsom are substantial organisations serving significant populations (81,000 and 24,000 people respectively). This sort of size has provided opportunities for skill differentiation, shared management infrastructure and economies of scale. A more modest example is the North Hillingdon PMS Pilot, where three small, previously separate, practices have come together to better serve a locality.

One of the defining characteristics of PMS has been the entry of NHS trusts into territory hitherto the exclusive domain of the independent contractor. This has led to the development of a number of innovative organisational models and some distinct benefits for patients. Tim Crossley has described how a community trust can directly provide primary care services, offering a salaried option to, sometimes beleaguered, single-handed practitioners. This may offer PCTs a strategy to retain some of the GPs they risk losing.

The Isleworth and Edith Cavell pilots have set up new primary care teams from scratch to meet needs persistently unmet through GMS. In these latter cases, patients have voted with their feet – both pilots filled their lists quickly. It would also appear that this model of care allows better integration with local community groups. Focus groups at each have endorsed the services as distinctly better in this regard than 'traditional' general practice.

A key feature of PMS has been the rise of the salaried GP. The national evaluation team suggests that this type of post may well assist with the recruitment crisis facing primary care. While the average salary of £44,674 is some way below the average intended net income of a full-time GMS GP, this appears to be compensated for through a significant package of other employment benefits. Eighty-five per cent of sites were satisfied with the quality of their applicants, and recruitment success was similar to that achieved by inner city practices generally.[14]

Our case studies raised an issue: the trade-off between autonomy and the need for managerial control. While many salaried GPs may enjoy the ability to focus on their clinical work, they will not have the same power to determine the running of the practice. However, our case studies and the evaluation of nurse-led pilots also suggested that community trusts may lack the managerial responsiveness necessary within a primary care setting. In these circumstances, salaried GPs may face the worst of all worlds – no managerial control, and little support either. Why is this? Certainly, community trusts faced steep learning curves as they entered an unfamiliar world; teething troubles were to be expected. However, it also speaks volumes about the ability of large organisations to react quickly to operational requirements. PCTs should think carefully when inheriting such schemes. Determining an appropriate level of managerial delegation and autonomy to practice level should be an early task.

Interestingly, both trust-led pilots have experienced significant staff turnover. Is this a sign that something is wrong? Probably not. Trust-led practices offer organisational stability and an infrastructure that will endure, whatever the personal fortunes of the staff employed within them. Contrast this to the traditional small practice: the retirement, illness, death, or other removal of the GP can be catastrophic to service continuity. Trust-led pilots offer a berth to clinical staff that does not have to be a commitment for life. This is a significant strength, particularly for the inner city. Of course, set against this, patients want personal continuity of care. Are trust-led pilots tantamount to an acceptance that, for some areas, this is now an unachievable aspiration?

PMS and the modernisation of primary care

'Modernisation' has become the mantra of this Government but, in the context of primary care, what does it mean? From the raft of policy statements and the utterances of Ministers it would appear that 'modern' primary care is bound up with an end to professional demarcations, the delivery of services that are responsive to the needs of individual patients and, above all, rapid and comprehensive access for patients.

Within this context, the early days of PMS should encourage the Government. Progress has been made across all of these fronts. Of course, none of these objectives are achieved only through PMS; many GMS practices might, with justification, claim that they too have made strides in the right direction. However, it seems plausible that PMS makes 'modernisation' more likely. In part, the reason for this is straightforward: the application process to join the scheme requires compliance with centrally articulated objectives. Potential pilots have to live up to these expectations.

However, structural issues may also make PMS a more suitable vehicle than the current GMS. For example, the focus of GMS remuneration on the individual GP rather than the team inhibits a radical review of skill mix. The broad application of capitation encourages some GPs to maintain high patient lists while offering a limited range of services. However, PMS mechanisms are by no means perfect. The application of funding can be 'clunky' – the rapid growth of both of the new practice pilots in our evaluation was not matched by a smooth increase in resources. The transfer of funds nationally between GMS and PMS budgets is complex and infrequent. More flexibility will be required for PMS to operate to maximum effectiveness.

The shifting of the PMS contract to PCTs increases the likelihood that local service development will be integrated across the previously impermeable boundaries of primary, community and hospital care. However, anomalies still exist in the commissioning of primary care. First and second wave pilots can still elect to keep their contracts with the local health authority. Pilots that are directly provided by PCTs themselves must be commissioned by their responsible health authority. With the number of health authorities set to reduce to 30 and their role to become overtly strategic, this appears a bizarre residual role that health authorities will find hard to discharge.

PMS pilots – the future?

From small beginnings, PMS pilots have grown in number and in significance. They have also continued to cause controversy within the medical profession. This should not be surprising. PMS can be characterised as an anti-monopoly measure: the monopoly of provision of primary care by independently contracted GPs has been broken by the introduction of new provider organisations, most noticeably NHS trusts and PCTs; the 'corporate' monopoly of the medical profession to negotiate terms with government has been sidestepped by local service agreements; and, lastly, the monopoly of doctors in the leadership role within primary care has been challenged by the development of new professional roles, most noticeably the 'nurse-led' PMS pilots. In a more fundamental sense, PMS is changing what it means to be a doctor. One of the essences of a profession lies in access to specialist knowledge;[15] increasingly, both this knowledge and the technical skills are held by nurses (among others).

Local contracting is now a key policy theme of the Labour Government. Personal dental services pilots were introduced at the same time as PMS pilots. The Health and Social Care Act 2001 has now extended local contracting to pharmaceutical services.

Whether the local contracting movement will galvanise the public–private partnerships announced by Tony Blair is moot. PMS pilots can, in theory, be managed by limited companies. However, in practice few of this type exist and the political barriers to entry seem high. Nevertheless, 'PMS Plus' pilots more easily allow the blurring of the private–NHS boundary. Tim Richardson and Andrew Roscoe described a nascent Health Maintenance Organisation with a complex mix of NHS and private providers. Certainly, local pharmaceutical services (LPS) pilots present clear opportunities for 'bodies corporate' to extend into NHS provision beyond the dispensing of medicines.

It has become a cliché to liken PMS to the fundholding flagship of the previous government. Both provided outlets for the entrepreneurial. Both catalysed unforeseen changes within the health service. PCGs and PCTs represented an attempt to universalise the best aspects of fundholding. In the same way, the work of the pilots described here looks set to join the mainstream of primary care.

References

1   Lewis R, Gillam S, Gosden T, Sheaff R. Who contracts for primary care? *Journal of Public Health Medicine* 1999; 21 (4): 367–72.

2   Sheaff R, Lloyd-Kendall A. Principal–agent relationships in general practice: the first wave of English personal medical services pilot contracts. *Journal of Health Services Research and Policy* 2000; 5 (3): 156–63.

3   Walsh N, André C, Barnes M, Huntington J, Rogers H, Baines D. Accountability, integration and responsiveness. In: *National evaluation of first wave NHS personal medical services pilots: integrated interim report from four research projects.* Manchester: NPCRDC, 2000.

4   Lewis R, Gillam S, editors. *Transforming primary care – personal medical services in the new NHS.* London: King's Fund, 1999.

5   Walsh N. Learning from evaluation of PMS pilots. Speech to NHS Confederation Conference, 5 July 2001, Manchester.

6   Steiner A, Campbell S, Robison J, Webb D, Sculpher M, Richards S, Roland M. Quality of care in PMS. In: *National evaluation of first wave NHS personal medical services pilots: integrated interim report from four research projects.* Manchester: NPCRDC, 2000.

7   Steiner A, Campbell S, Robison J, Webb D, Sculpher M, Richards S, Roland M. Quality of care in PMS. In: *National evaluation of first wave NHS personal medical services pilots: integrated interim report from four research projects.* Manchester: NPCRDC, 2000.

8   Carter Y, Curtis S, Harding G, Maguire A, Meads G, Riley A, Ross T, Underwood M. Addressing inequalities. In: *National evaluation of first wave NHS personal medical services pilots: integrated interim report from four research projects.* Manchester: NPCRDC, 2000.

9   Jenkins C, Lewis R. Reducing inequality. In: Lewis R, Gillam S, editors. *Transforming primary care – personal medical services in the new NHS.* London: King's Fund, 1999.

10 Lewis R, Gillam, S. What seems to be the trouble? *Health Service Journal* 2000; 110: 28–30.

11 Walsh N, Allen L, Baines D, Barnes M. *A first year report of the personal medical services (PMS) pilots in England.* Birmingham: HSMC, 1999.

12 Chapple A, Rogers A, Macdonald W, Sergison M. Patients' perceptions of changing professional boundaries and the future of 'nurse-led' services. *Primary Health Care Research and Development* 2000; 1: 51–9.

13 Chapple A, Rogers A, Macdonald W, Sergison M. Patients' perceptions of changing professional boundaries and the future of 'nurse-led' services. *Primary Health Care Research and Development* 2000 1: 51–9.

14 Williams J, Petchey R, Gosden T, Leese B, Sibbald B. A profile of PMS salaried GP contracts and their impact on recruitment. *Family Practice* 2001; 18 (3): 283–7.

15 Freidson E. *The profession of medicine: a study of the sociology of applied knowledge.* New York: Harper and Row, 1970.